Praise from the experts

'Let thy medicine be thy food and th[...] ...naps even truer today than when it was coine[...] ...e than 2000 years ago. The relationship between diet [...] an important one, and women in particular, want to know [...] they can do to reduce their risk. Taking information that is often confusing and contradictory, Dr. Robert Pendergrast has written a book that is practical, highly informative and easy to understand. Any woman who is looking to give herself 'an edge' against cancer should read this book.

— Tieraona Low Dog, M.D., Director of the Fellowship,
Arizona Center for Integrative Medicine

Robert Pendergrast has written more than a good book on nutritional prevention of cancer. *Breast Cancer: Reduce Your Risk with Foods You Love* is a model for a new way for Americans to think about health, whether cancer, heart disease or any other serious health issue. Instead of hoping to find it early and treat it, Robert points out the way to never have to find it at all!

— Dr. Roger Jahnke, CEO of Health Action Synergies,
author of *The Healer Within*

Correctly noting that 'unfortunately, nutritional illiteracy is still commonplace among doctors,' Robert Pendergrast immediately joins the ranks of the literati with *Breast Cancer: Reduce Your Risk with Foods You Love*. This easily accessible gem will become an invaluable resource not only for women but for the men and children in their lives because it offers sane nutritional information that will likely reduce the risk of other malignancies as well. This book will find its place right between *Foods That Fight Cancer* and *The Cancer-Fighting Kitchen* on my office bookshelf, readily available to recommend to all the patients that I counsel. Thank you, Dr. Pendergrast, for presenting such a wealth of information in a practical guidebook so easy to digest and absorb!

> — Donald I. Abrams, M.D., Integrative Oncology, University of California, San Francisco, Osher Center for Integrative Medicine; Chief, Hematology-Oncology, San Francisco General Hospital; Professor of Clinical Medicine, University of California, San Francisco

As a two-time breast cancer survivor, I will strongly encourage my friends and professional contacts to read and put into practice Dr. Pendergrast's book, *Breast Cancer: Reduce Your Risk with Foods You Love.* Not only are the guidelines for good nutrition in this book a necessity if I am to remain cancer free, women also can use it as a guide to maintain optimal overall health.

> — Nita Zachow, Executive Committee, Breast Cancer Prevention Coalition, Patient Advisory Committee, Medical College of Georgia

In an elegantly simple and personal style, Dr. Robert Pendergrast has wrapped a wealth of information into *Breast Cancer: Reduce Your Risk with Foods You Love.* His message is the same one I have been teaching for years: Nutrition is the key to disease prevention. If all women were to follow this guide to optimum breast health, it would mark a turning point in the war on breast cancer, from treatment to primary prevention. I will recommend this book to patients, colleagues, and friends.

> — Andrew Weil, M.D., author of *Eating Well for Optimum Health, Healthy Aging,* Founder/Director of the Arizona Center for Integrative Medicine

BREAST CANCER

Reduce Your Risk
with Foods You Love

BREAST CANCER

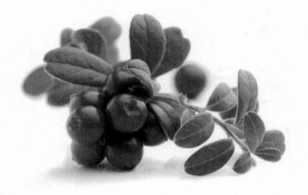

Reduce Your Risk
with Foods You Love

Robert Pendergrast, MD

Breast Cancer: Reduce Your Risk with Foods You Love
By Robert Pendergrast, MD, MPH
Copyright © 2011 Robert Pendergrast

Published by

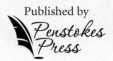
Penstokes
Press

Cover and Interior Design: NZ Graphics
Editing: Danielle Wong Moores and John Maling

Library of Congress Control Number: 2010923246
ISBN: 978-0-9844769-0-9

1. Breast Cancer   2. Cancer Prevention   3. Nutrition   4. Health

First Edition Printed in Canada

Books may be purchased by contacting the publisher, Penstokes Press at:
www.PenstokesPress.com

Dedicated to the memory of
Dianne Lyles: July 7, 1947 – September 5, 2005

Table of Contents

Introduction

A few years ago, a large hospital system placed a full-page newspaper advertisement. The headline read:

You Can't Prevent Breast Cancer

My reaction to those words was immediate and outraged. It is such judgments that create the sense of fear and dread among women. It pervades the thinking of many, drowning out any discussion about real strategies intended to reduce risk. Here was a medical system promoting that very assumption!

Having gone to great lengths to study and apply the latest research on cancer risk reduction through nutrition, I knew that the words in the headline were not true. I also knew from my personal and professional encounters that if I asked the question, "Is breast cancer preventable?" at the local shopping mall, very few women would be able to answer a ringing and confident, "Yes!" The pervasive fear, the fatalistic hoping that one might have "good luck" and avoid the disease, has in part been the result of the emphasis of doctors and hospitals embodied in that headline.

The medical establishment, including research institutions, professional medical societies, hospitals and the pharmaceutical industry for the past 100 years, has been focused almost exclusively on treatment instead of prevention. And conventional medical education for doctors in training has, to date, been almost devoid of emphasis on the power of foods to prevent disease.[1] The widespread cultural fatalism about breast cancer is, in part, the result of the relentless emphasis by the medical establishment on treatment and cure *to the exclusion of a prevention message.*

To see that same system exploiting that fear by actually claiming the disease was not preventable was, and is, too much for me to be quiet about. I knew, as many do, that prevention for any single individual, and

1

risk reduction for the population at large, was achievable with a diet of healing foods that are not only powerful but delicious and affordable!

Treatment is Good . . . Prevention is Better.

Why do you suppose a hospital would place an ad like that in the first place? The body of the ad went on to explain that even though this very scary situation was not preventable, it was treatable, and that this particular health system had in fact the best treatment options available. It sounded so reassuring.

Don't get me wrong; I am all for the best treatment of disease, and I support research into cancer treatment that will save the lives of cancer patients. We are making progress. But I was upset, even angry, when that advertisement glared out at me. Because I knew it left out exactly the information that women need to make the choices that will reduce their risk of getting breast cancer in the first place.

The best "treatment" is never having the disease in the first place. That half-truth in bold letters in the local paper could well have reinforced the unspoken fears of countless women who read it that day: "I am helpless, I am afraid, and all I can do is wait and hope for the best." The gut reaction I had to that half-truth propelled me into the mission of writing this book.

Breast Cancer the Home-Wrecker

In 2005, Dianne Lyles was dying. Barely 58 years old, she had been fighting breast cancer for over 10 years. With multiple metastases after her bone marrow transplant, she was weakening rapidly and was in constant pain.

I was reminded of the very personal way that breast cancer touches families when visiting Dianne in her home in a small town in southern Georgia. Women like Dianne are the cornerstone of family life in their communities. She was the only child of hardworking parents—a farmer and a schoolteacher. Later she became a gifted teacher herself, known throughout the county for her work with elementary grades, high school music, drama, and literary competitions, as well as private music lessons.

More than a few of my medical students were awed to find out that I knew "Mrs. Lyles" who had been their favorite teacher in high school. And yet they also painfully knew that she had retired early from teaching because of illness, and that her gifts would never be known by another generation of students.

Not only had she touched families throughout the area with her teaching, she also brought up three children and supported her husband as he worked long hours running the family business. The cancer that she spent years fighting not only weakened her, it also diminished her contributions in all those areas. And that same fight also affected the next generation, as her daughter postponed going to college and then eventually quit her job in order to move back home and care for her mother in her final year.

The last time I saw Dianne in her home, she was surrounded by family: her adult children, and two grandchildren who would be too young to ever remember their grandmother as they grew up. Years earlier, at the birth of her youngest child, my wife had gone home with her from the hospital to help in the household. Though they were cousins, not siblings, they grew up in the loyalty of a small family like sisters. Now, at this difficult transition, she was back again, helping in whatever small ways she could. As for me, having married into this close family, it was a time of intense awareness, observation and reflection.

The impact of breast cancer on the usual rhythm of a family history was striking. Dianne spent the last 10 years of her life, in her 40s and 50s, preoccupied with cancer treatments. Not to say she didn't get anything else done—the woman was an incredible multi-tasker. How much energy and time did that take away from her family life? Or, from the care she could have given her elderly mother? From the richness of watching her children marry? The anticipation and joy of watching her grandchildren grow and learn? The students that would never be able to say she was the best teacher they ever had? And, from the rewards of retirement and travels with her first love, the sweetheart she'd married barely out of school herself?

Not only was she robbed of those treasures, her family and community were robbed of her place at that time of her life.

The Long View from Childhood

As a pediatrician with years of practice experience, something else caught my eye in that room full of family members—her granddaughter, a toddler.

This child would remember her grandmother only in pictures and stories. But someday, I knew from experience, a doctor would ask her about a family history of breast cancer. Perhaps that doctor would then teach the young woman about breast self-exams. Or years later perhaps, order a mammogram, knowing that her grandmother had died young with the disease.

As a pediatrician, and director of adolescent medicine training programs in two medical schools, I had spent countless hours talking with kids and teens about nutrition and health. I had many times been the first doctor to teach a teenage girl about breast health and how to do a breast self-exam.

Most pediatricians are passionate about prevention and health promotion. I was no exception but had taken that passion a step further than most of my colleagues. After my residency and fellowship I went back to school (much to my wife's dismay) to get a public health degree from Johns Hopkins. By the time I received the Master of Public Health degree, my medical vision had been expanded beyond the individual patient to the impact that I could make on the community, the nation, and the world.

When I looked with pediatric public health eyes at that little toddler, and I thought about the half-truth in the newspaper ad that said breast cancer cannot be prevented, my mission was born. *Breast Cancer: Reduce Your Risk with Foods You Love* is my attempt to spread the word to as many women and young girls as possible. By doing so, their breasts can be kept healthy through healing foods. As they enter their 50s, 60s and beyond, they can continue to give and receive the treasures of relationships, family and community life in towns small and large.

But as I look around, some days I feel I am fighting an uphill battle. The prevailing sentiment these days is "hope for a cure." There's not much talk about prevention. But there is much talk about treatments, and a great sense of fatalism and hoping for "good luck" among women.

That sentiment is reinforced in subtle ways repeatedly in our medically dependent society.

Early Detection vs. Prevention

You can see it play out all around you. In grocery stores, public service announcements printed on shopping bags and at checkouts say "Early Detection: Your Best Protection." Of all places, a grocery store would be a great place to say, "Great Food Choices Available in the Produce Section—Scientifically Supported Real Prevention."

Please understand: there is no magical diet that can 100 percent guarantee that a woman will not get breast cancer. But there *are* though, specific choices of foods that over time will move a woman out of the group called "more likely to get breast cancer" and *into* the group called "not as likely to get breast cancer." That's terrific news, because anyone can do it. The other good news: eating to prevent breast cancer is also excellent prevention for heart disease (the leading killer of women), and similarly reduces the risk of prostate cancer (in men), and other cancers.

Risk Reduction: You're Always Either 0% or 100%

What does *risk reduction* really mean? All of the prevention messages in books, billboards, magazines and the airwaves are an effort to reduce your statistical probability of getting a "bad" outcome like cancer, heart disease, or diabetes.

The classic, best-known example is to stop smoking. For decades we have known that cigarette smoking is the most important preventable cause of lung cancer, and people who stop smoking begin to reduce their risk immediately. Granted, there are plenty of cigarette smokers who "dodge the bullet" and make it all the way through life without cancer. And we know that there are many people who are diagnosed with lung cancer who never smoked a cigarette and never lived with a smoker. Though there is overlap in both directions (smokers who stay healthy and non-smokers who get sick), it is not a random process. We, and you, can still make sense of risk reduction.

For any one individual at a point in time, you either have cancer (100 percent risk), or you don't (0 percent risk). When a person moves through life and never gets the disease, prevention has worked for that individual. Because that is not a guaranteed outcome, let's look at risk reduction instead—how to move yourself into a group more likely to get that 100 percent prevention outcome.

You Get to Choose Your Chances of Getting There

Imagine a long line of people waiting their turn to get into a theater that has two movies. When the customers get to the front of the line, the ticket taker sends all the smokers into the movie called *High Probability of Getting Sick,* and the non-smokers are assigned to the other movie, *Low Probability of Getting Sick.* Now put yourself in the line approaching the ticket taker. Wouldn't you want to choose the *Low Probability of Getting Sick* movie versus the other?

Even though you know you still could become ill, you know your chances are better if you go with the low probability option. And you get to stay with that group of people by behaving in ways that reduce your risk—by stopping smoking.

You will have the same experience by reading and using *Breast Cancer: Reduce your Risk with Foods You Love.* You get to stay with the "low-risk," low probability group by eating in specific ways that have been studied and shown to reduce risk of breast cancer.

Take Action . . . Don't Wait for More Studies

The other important concept I would like to clarify here is the concept of the amount of evidence required to recommend a particular medical intervention. In the past decade, doctors have become very fond of practicing "evidence-based medicine." This means only techniques and treatments are recommended that have shown a positive benefit in randomized clinical trials. Preferably where the investigators and patients were blinded to whether they were getting a "real" intervention or a placebo.

This is considered the gold standard in evidence-based medical practice. It has been whimsically pointed out that there are no random-ized clinical trials of the health benefits of wearing a parachute when you jump out of an airplane. Such a study does not need to be done, nor will you get any volunteers. And on the opposite end of the continuum, how much evidence of benefit will you require to be shown before you recommend a medical service that has virtually no potential to do harm to a patient?

If a treatment has significant potential toxicity, I had better prove beyond all doubt that it works before I recommend it to my patients. But if the preventive treatment is benign (foods) and the problem is serious (cancer), rational thinking gives the go-ahead to that approach even if scientific evidence is small. Critics of this book may look at my food recommendations for preventing breast cancer and say there are not enough studies to claim that these recommendations are scientifically valid. That is shortsighted and lacks common sense.

My response is simple: if there is any evidence showing that a food can reduce breast cancer risk, and the food itself has minimal potential for harm, then we should be recommending that food. Breast cancer is too prevalent and too serious to wait any longer for randomized clinical trials of foods. The information on foods I present and highly recommend is backed by scientific studies of humans and under laboratory conditions. If the evidence base is not as strong as some would like, let the scientists argue. In the meantime, I am confident that all of the recommendations in this book will reduce your disease risk.

There's More to Health than Food

It is not an accident that I choose to focus your attention on food choices as your key to reducing breast cancer risk. And also, if you were to come to me in my office for a consultation and ask for tools to decrease that risk, we would cover more than just food choices.

My personal goal is for you to implement the program outlined in this book and believe it will make a huge difference in prevention. I also hope you will use this as a starting point for other health promoting choices.

In our office consult, I would talk with you about at least seven distinct but interacting areas:

1. Herbal medicine and nutritional supplements;
2. The use of stress reduction techniques such as conscious breathing and mental imagery;
3. Your exercise habits;
4. The role of physical medicine and manipulation such as massage or osteopathic manipulation;
5. Opening the flow of energy in the body through disciplines such as Qigong (chee-gung), acupuncture, or Healing Touch;

6. Your spiritual life and sense of meaning in the world; and

7. The environment with which you surround yourself.

It is probably no surprise to you that I learned little if any of that in medical school. My medical school training and my specialty training in pediatrics was biomedical, based on a model of diagnosing a disease and eliminating it. This biomedical model has worked quite well over the past 100 years. It has produced amazing results in surgical repair, antimicrobial treatment for infections as simple as strep throat or as complex as HIV/AIDS; insulin to protect against the ravages of diabetes, and the list goes on.

With all our advances in technological medicine, we often succumb to the temptation to see human beings as machines. Find the broken part and either fix it or replace it. People are much more wonderful and complex than automobile engines. And unlike an auto engine, a human being who has a broken part replaced may continue to feel ill. I cannot count the number of times I have sat in an exam room with a patient and heard these words: "My doctor says that there's nothing wrong with me. All the lab tests are normal, so why do I still feel terrible every day?"

If we define health as simply the inability of our tests and x-rays to find an abnormality, then it's no wonder doctors are at a loss to explain why you may feel badly. A better way would be for doctors to embrace the following concept:

Health is a state of complete physical, mental and social well-being and not merely the absence of disease or infirmity.[2]

These clear words are from the preamble to the constitution of the World Health Organization, unchanged since 1948! With them we can give some hope to patients who know they are not well even when there is not a diagnosed disease.

As doctors, we can start helping our patients acquire health by attending to those seven areas I listed above; this is the foundation of prevention and wellness.

Optimism Starts Today

Can you prevent breast cancer? Absolutely! By following the guidelines in this book throughout their lives, women can reduce their risk of the disease. You can take control of your health by controlling your lifestyle and food choices on a day-to-day basis.

I want you to find this book to be empowering for you, giving you the knowledge you need to sift through all the information and choices you face, and ending the day with hope and optimism for the future, for yourself, for your daughters, and for your families.

PART 1

General Guidelines for Cancer Prevention

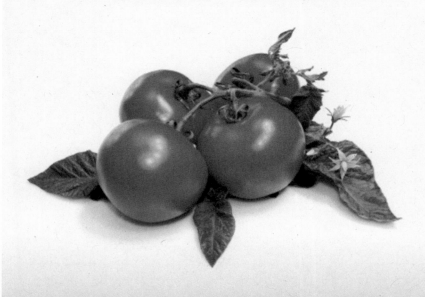

CHAPTER 1
Paint a Colorful Diet

In Part 2, I will give you considerable detail on 10 specific foods that I believe are among your strongest breast cancer prevention allies. But if you go straight to those chapters, you may miss an important concept: it is the overall pattern, mix and variety of your diet that is the most important food factor in cancer prevention. Your best habit for cancer risk reduction day by day is to eat a large variety of healthy foods instead of focusing on just one or two in the "Top 10" list. A large amount of good science links a diet high in fresh fruits and vegetables with decreased cancer risk across the board.

It's What's on Your Plate that Matters

Most of what is on your plate at every meal should be from plants, and very colorful ones at that. Darkly pigmented fruits such as blueberries, blackberries and raspberries are antioxidant powerhouses. Colorful vegetables such as carrots, sweet potatoes or red cabbage and vegetables with dark green leaves like kale, chard or spring mix for salads are great. The *Brassica* family of vegetables, well represented by broccoli, cabbage, cauliflower, kale, bok choy and brussel sprouts, are especially important in reducing risks of cancer of the breast, colon, lung and stomach. It's best to enjoy them fresh and not overcooked. I also encourage people to buy organically grown produce whenever possible, to minimize the body's exposure to agricultural chemical residue.

13

The evidence supporting a diet high in a wide variety of vegetables and fruits as a key cancer prevention strategy is well established; it is widely known among nutrition scientists and journalists covering such topics, but not widely known in the general public.

> **Next time you are at a party, try opening a conversation with, "Say, do you know what percentage of cancer cases is estimated to be preventable by dietary choices?"**

The American Institute for Cancer Research (AICR) and the World Cancer Research Fund have jointly published an expert report, most recently updated and modified in 2007 that consistently links dietary choices high in vegetable and fruits with lower cancer risk. The consensus opinion of the report is that one-third of all cancers are preventable by diet. This is a globally consistent finding, not just in the U.S. or in industrialized nations. It is also a finding applicable to a variety of cancers in many parts of the body. This implies that regardless of their diversity, a wide variety of cancers are, at their root, partially dependent on environmental factors for their genesis and propagation. Conversely, a healthy food environment can and does protect against cancer's development in several different body areas and organ systems.[1]

On the other hand, there have been articles published in the recent American scientific literature that concluded that no statistical link has been found between vegetable and fruit intake and breast cancer risk.[2] With all due respect to the meticulous work done by those authors and their scientific credentials, I believe the problem with their conclusion is what Michael Pollan refers to in his excellent and thought-provoking book, *In Defense of Food*, as "the elephant in the room."[3]

The elephant in the room is this: Despite small differences in vegetable and fruit intake, almost everyone in that study was still eating the *standard American diet.* That distinctly American way of eating has evolved over the past 50 years so that, compared to other countries, it is:

- Very high in sugars and refined carbohydrates;
- High in saturated fats, inflammatory vegetable oils and trans-fats;
- High in chemical additives and preservatives; and
- Low in fresh vegetables and fruit.

Dietary differences between groups in the negative studies are simply not profound enough to demonstrate a difference in outcomes. I believe from the evidence I have seen that prevention of breast cancer is possible, and that increased vegetable and fruit intake is part of that strategy. However, it will take more than "tweaking" our usual dietary habits in America.

Dr. David Heber has written about the powerful potential of phytochemicals from a colorful variety of plant foods in his excellent book, *What Color is Your Diet?* Dr. Heber points out that cancer is a disease of DNA damage in human cells.[4] His research shows that antioxidants from a plateful of colorful vegetables and fruits protect against DNA damage to your cells. It's not hard to connect the dots and say without any doubt that eating his colorful, plant-based diet will protect against cancer. The evidence is inescapable.

Phytochemicals: Nature's Pharmaceutical Prevention Formula

Phytochemicals were not recognized a generation ago, but now we know that chemical compounds plants produce to protect themselves from oxidative damage to DNA also protect the humans who eat them. Groups of chemicals—such as flavonoids and polyphenols—are examples of phytochemicals with cancer-protective mechanisms which are widely found in nature.

> **Accumulating evidence regarding the protective effect of vegetables and fruits points to the role of phytochemicals, more than vitamins and minerals, as the protective superstars in plants.**

The presence of this enormous array of chemical compounds in plants, which are still being discovered and clarified, brings to mind two important observations.

First, our best protection is in whole foods and not supplements, extracts or pills. The history of "nutritionism" (as Pollan calls our pseudo-religious faith in the *reductionistic* science of finding the "single right ingredient" in foods that accounts for their health benefits) is littered with scientific shortsightedness and omissions. Never believe that a pill, or a single set of nutrient extracts from foods, will be able to convey the same protective benefit to you as the whole foods (vegetables and fruits) themselves.

Second, reflect on the superabundance of compounds in edible plants on this planet that protect human health. I cannot help but find myself in awe and wonder at the wisdom of the created order of things; that nature's pharmacy is so generous in making disease prevention available to our species.

By now, you may be getting excited about vegetables and fruits, but there are already accountants out there reading this who are saying, "But how many servings per day are enough, and how big is a serving anyway?" I recommend nine servings of vegetables and fruits (combined) per day. Serving sizes are typically a

> **Getting to the holy grail of nine servings is easier than you might have imagined, since these serving sizes are smaller than we are accustomed to seeing in our oversized serving world of the early 21st century.**

half-cup of cooked, raw or frozen vegetables and fruit, and one cup of leafy vegetables.

Good Fats, Bad Fats

Another very important part of your colorful and varied food choices for preventing cancer is your selection of oils and fats. A study in the *Journal of the National Cancer Institute* in 1995 showed an increased risk in breast cancer for women who ate margarine, and a reduced risk of breast cancer for those who consumed olive oil instead of margarine.[5] My conclusion on reviewing all the data on fats is that your risk of cancer can be reduced by:

- Avoiding all trans-fats (margarine, vegetable shortening and any packaged baked goods with the words "hydrogenated" or "partially hydrogenated" on the label);
- Increasing the use of extra-virgin olive oil in cooking, salad dressings, etc; and by
- Increasing your omega-3 fat intake through oily fish such as salmon or sardines, or taking a fish oil capsule.

At the risk of getting too technical, I think it's important for you to understand about how oils and fats are classified so that you will have the basic information needed to sort through your dietary choices. Because of the current bad reputation of fats generally, I feel I need to give some reassuring comments about fats in general.

With health claims on food labels everywhere trumpeting phrases like "low fat!" and "no cholesterol!" and "no trans-fats!," one gets the sense we have never recovered from the fat phobia that has permeated nutrition science for much of the last 30 years. Let me be clear:

Fat is not the enemy!
(Nor are carbohydrates the enemy—more about that later).

We all need fat in the diet, and the world nutrition literature is clear that the human organism not only can thrive on a fairly high percentage of fat in foods, but also requires fats and oils to be consumed regularly for optimal health. But are there good and bad fats? In nature, the answer is probably no, it's more a matter of their proportions in the diet.

Types of Fats and Where They Are Found

Fats naturally occur in three forms: saturated, mono-unsaturated and poly-unsaturated. The three forms differ according to the number of double bonds between carbon atoms in the long chains that characterize the basic component of fats, the so-called "fatty acids."

Saturated fats have no double bonds; mono-unsaturated fats have one double bond; and poly-unsaturated fats have more than one double bond. Foods (plant or animal) typically contain a mix of these, but in general, animal products are higher in saturated fats than are vegetable products.

Including a variety of foods in the diet is therefore important. Fish for example, are especially high in a type of essential poly-unsaturated fat called omega-3 fatty acid. On the other hand, olive oil is the quintessential source of mono-unsaturated fats, also important to our health.

All of these fats are *necessary* to our health in their own way, but the modern Western diet has developed into a pattern of excesses in certain types of fats and deficiencies in others. These excesses and deficiencies are leading to health problems in our population.

Avoid Excess on Either End of the Saturation Spectrum

Most preventive cardiologists will tell you that a standard strategy for reducing cholesterol and thereby reducing the risk of heart disease is to cut the amount of saturated fat in the diet (translate that to mean less meat and less dairy). A few studies however, have suggested there is actually very little scientific support for this approach.

On the other end of the saturation spectrum, our standard Western diet gives us an excess of a particular class of poly-unsaturated fatty acids called omega-6. Omega-6 fatty acids, primarily found in vegetable oils, are essential for life, but when their intake far exceeds that of the omega-3s, excessive and unneeded inflammation results in the body.

Inflammation is at the root of many, if not most, of the chronic diseases that tend to beset Americans as we move into our older years. A dietary approach to fat intake that has gained increasing scientific support as a preventive strategy against chronic disease is:

- Eat *more* foods containing omega-3s (fish or flax seed for example), and,
- Eat *less* food containing omega-6s (liquid vegetable oils used in cooking, salad dressings and baked products, such as corn oil, peanut oil, soy oil, and safflower and sunflower oils).

While we clearly need to increase our omega-3 intake (by eating fish) and decrease our omega-6 intake (by using less vegetable oil), a simple way to approach that would be to follow Michael Pollan's dictum. It is,

Eat foods

rather than eat highly processed foods, which are more likely to contain high concentrations of omega-6 vegetable oils.

You can feel pretty comfortable about your natural fat intake by eating fish twice a week and simply staying away from foods that have a label and list of ingredients.

You've no doubt heard about trans-fats. What about them? How do they fit into the structure of a healthy diet?

Trans-Fats: We Actually Thought These Were Better for Us

For the most part, trans-fats are an artificial species, created by the process of hydrogenating (or partially hydrogenating) poly-unsaturated vegetable oils. The advantage to food manufacturers is that the process creates a solid spreadable fat like butter out of liquid vegetable oil which is known as margarine. And it is less expensive than butter.

Hydrogenation and partial hydrogenation also increase the shelf life of those processed foods by making it less likely that the fats contained in the foods will oxidize and cause the product to become rancid. While nutrition science in the 1960s thought it was doing us a favor by serving us margarine instead of butter, research since then has made it clear that trans-fats are actually pro-inflammatory and represent a great risk for worsening cholesterol levels and heart disease. Margarine does not belong on your table.

Also alarming are data from a European study published in June 2008 in the *American Journal of Epidemiology*. The research demonstrated that women with higher levels of trans-fats in the blood were more likely to have breast cancer.[6] It seems prudent at this time to avoid all trans-fats by carefully reading package labels. If the words "hydrogenated" or "partially hydrogenated" oils appear on the label, do not purchase or consume that product, even if the front of the package boasts "no trans-fats."

Good Fats from Real Foods You Love

Getting healthy fats into the diet is easier than you might think. Some quick suggestions: Walnuts on your cereal or oatmeal in the morning; a can of sardines on wheat crackers with salsa for lunch; or wild Alaskan salmon for dinner. Have fish twice a week. Use extra virgin olive oil as your preferred cooking oil. When the flavor of the olive oil is too much, use expeller-pressed organic (non-GMO) canola oil.

Moving On to Blood Sugar

We have so far emphasized the importance of abundant and varied vegetables and fruits in your diet as a cancer prevention strategy.

(Sounds familiar, doesn't it? Was it something your mother said about eating those vegetables?) And, equally important is the role of healthy oils in preventing inflammation and its disease consequences. I also believe we have enough good science now to be confident in recommending a *low glycemic index diet* that is good for cancer prevention.

You probably never heard your mother say anything about the glycemic index of your food, but in the last 20 years or so, data favorable to the concept from a nutritional viewpoint have been steadily accumulating on this topic. In a nutshell, this means focusing on getting your carbohydrates from vegetables and whole grains instead of starches and refined grains. It also means getting the largest part of your daily carbohydrate intake from non-starchy vegetables and fruits.

What is the glycemic index, and why should you care?

The glycemic index refers to the ability of a specific food to raise blood sugar levels—how high and for how long. Pure sugar (glucose) is given a score of 100. And just like golf, in the case of the glycemic index as it relates to your health, a low score wins. Foods (and drinks) that have a glycemic index of less than 55 are considered to have a *low glycemic index*. You generally want to stay in that low range. Why? Spikes in blood sugar are a signal to the body that sugar levels need to be brought down by being transformed and stored (as triglycerides— fats that eventually are stored around your middle). The hormone that your body calls on to down-regulate those blood sugar spikes is insulin.

Insulin is a very powerful hormone, and over time, prolonged elevations in insulin levels (necessary to keep your blood sugar in check) are a major risk factor for cardiovascular disease and cancers. Insulin is a tumor growth promoter when its levels stay on the high side. Most likely it's why people with Type 2 diabetes (a condition of *insulin resistance*, by cells failing to allow insulin to introduce sugar through their cellular membranes) have higher rates of cancer than the general population. That alone is a very important reason why you want to avoid high-glycemic foods that can cause frequent spikes in blood sugar (think sweets, flour and starch).

The glycemic index is also related to our old nemesis, excess inflammation. Recent research has shown that the overall *glycemic load* of foods (glycemic index of the food multiplied by the quantity of carbohydrate eaten) is related to chemical markers in the blood that indicate inflammation in the body.[7]

Is inflammation an independent risk factor for cancer? Mounting evidence indicates that the answer is yes. Cancers in numerous organ systems have been shown to be associated with chronic inflammation as a likely contributor to its development.[8]

A common theme you will find throughout the dietary recommendations in this book is that the healing foods recommended invariably reduce inflammation, or they replace an unhealthy food that is pro-inflammatory and therefore pro-cancer. Right now, add high glycemic index foods to your list of inflammatory foods that may promote cancer development.[9]

Whole Grains, Refined Carbohydrates, and the Glycemic Index

Does this mean that carbohydrates are the enemy? No. It means that a diet high in *refined* carbohydrates and low in whole grains is hazardous to your health. Sometimes, however, defining *whole grain* foods can be challenging. A stroll down the cereal aisle in your local supermarket will reveal a number of sugary breakfast cereals that make "whole grain" claims on their labels. How do you sort out what's whole grain and what's not?

A whole grain food, most purely defined, is one where you can still see the grain—it is not ground up. Rice counts as a whole grain, but only brown rice, because in white rice a large part of the grain has been polished away (the healthiest part).

Whole wheat bread, as it is found in grocery stores, does not count as a whole grain product because the grain has been ground into such fine flour that its glycemic index is virtually indistinguishable from white bread. (I still recommend whole wheat bread over white bread because it is higher in fiber and protein, and as long as it doesn't contain hydrogenated or partially hydrogenated vegetable oils).

Rolled oats (as granola or oatmeal for example) is a good example of a whole grain.

Does that mean you never eat bread or pasta? Of course not! And pasta if not overcooked can be a low glycemic index food. Just think of them as foods to eat in moderation, and always mix them with some healthy oil (like olive oil) and protein. The mixing of those foods lowers the glycemic index of the carbohydrate when eaten together with its partners in the mix.

Please enjoy grains without guilt or fear. The health benefits of whole grains are well known: they are one way to increase fiber in the diet. They reduce risk of colon cancer, can help to lower LDL cholesterol, reduce constipation and reduce risk of diverticular disease of the large intestine.

To briefly summarize how to eat a low glycemic index diet (which I believe is overall one of your best health-promoting dietary strategies):

- Decrease your intake of potatoes (sweet potatoes, however, are fine and have a naturally low glycemic index).
- Decrease your intake of breads and when you do eat them; choose coarse, stone-ground, whole grain breads.
- Choose breakfast cereals made from oats, barley and other whole grains (the longer the time needed to cook your oats the better; *instant* means high glycemic index).
- Keep your plate full of fresh fruits and vegetables.
- Choose brown rice or basmati rice.
- Pasta generally is a low glycemic index food and can be eaten in small to moderate quantities.

Think of these carbohydrate foods as always to be enjoyed mixed with healthy oils and some protein, because this slows the release of sugars into the bloodstream. A good example would be spaghetti with an olive oil pesto sauce and cottage or Romano cheese.

The Joy of Eating Good Food!

Remember, food is good! It is to be enjoyed and shared with gratitude with people you enjoy, in a relaxed atmosphere around the dinner table. The conversation at a healthy meal should not be about the health qualities of the food, but about the delicious tastes and aromas, and the shared life experiences of friends!

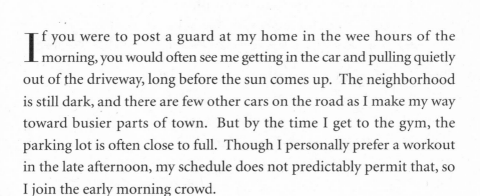

Chapter 2
Moderate Exercise

If you were to post a guard at my home in the wee hours of the morning, you would often see me getting in the car and pulling quietly out of the driveway, long before the sun comes up. The neighborhood is still dark, and there are few other cars on the road as I make my way toward busier parts of town. But by the time I get to the gym, the parking lot is often close to full. Though I personally prefer a workout in the late afternoon, my schedule does not predictably permit that, so I join the early morning crowd.

And what a crowd! By 6:00 a.m. most of the elliptical machines and treadmills are taken, guys in tank tops and big muscles are straining at the free weights, the morning basketball leagues are going strong, with "trash talk" echoing off the court, and people are swimming laps in the cool water. So while I may have been bleary eyed leaving the house and wondering what I am doing up so early, I am suddenly energized just walking into the place.

And I am inspired when I look around me at the others who have made that early morning commitment. Some are obviously in great shape, fit and trim. But some are older people, maybe walking with a post-operative limp around the indoor track. That "I'm not giving up" attitude inspires me. And some are very overweight and often struggling and out of breath as they keep moving, step after step. They keep showing up for exercise even knowing there are a few people in every gym who look down on overweight people with mean intolerance. I am especially inspired by that group, because they have decided to take action and make physical fitness a priority, "whatever it takes."

I do not know why all those people are at the gym, or what motivates them to brave the morning dark and cold; but . . .

> **I wonder if any of the women know that they are actively reducing their risk of breast cancer by staying physically active!**

Exercise: Healthy Prevention in Every Step

In late 20th century in America, economic changes resulted in a generally more sedentary population than had been seen in earlier generations. People more often used machines to do work they used to do by hand, and they used machines to carry them to places where they used to walk. As it became obvious to medical science that a sedentary lifestyle was a health hazard, the concept of aerobic exercise as a leisure activity became a cultural phenomenon in the 60s and 70s. That was thanks largely to Dr. Kenneth Cooper. Then a whole new industry of athletic shoes was born, and gyms became known as *health clubs*.

The common wisdom of the time was that this aerobic exercise was a benefit to cardiovascular health (which it is). But research since then has demonstrated convincingly that regular physical activity is associated with a large array of other health benefits, including lower rates of cancer.

The American Institute for Cancer Research updated its major report on cancer, nutrition and physical activity in 2007. The conclusion of the review of countless scientific papers by this major scientific body is that regular physical activity protects against several types of cancer: specifically, colon cancer, breast cancer (post-menopausal) and cancer of the uterus (endometrium). They noted that this reduction in risk is accounted for by the physical activity itself and not simply as a function of lower weight.

To be clear:

> **Increased physical activity reduces risk of cancer regardless of body weight.**

But since we know that obesity is itself also an independent risk factor for cancer, and that higher levels of physical activity are associated with less obesity, it also follows that regular physical activity reduces risk of cancers by the pathway of weight reduction.

Body Weight and Breast Cancer Risk

The relationship between weight and breast cancer is understood only in relationship to whether a woman is before or after menopause. Premenopausal breast cancer seems to be in many ways a different disease than post-menopausal breast cancer, and it has a different set of risk factors.

The data are clear that being overweight is a risk factor for post-menopausal breast cancer. A woman who carries more body fat than she needs is more likely to develop breast cancer after menopause. This is at least partly related to the ability of fatty tissues to increase the overall levels of estrogen in a woman's body. The activity of an enzyme called aromatase is higher in fatty tissues, and one of the functions of aromatase is to convert other circulating steroids in the bloodstream to estrogen.

In summary, the chain of events works like this:

The higher a woman's lifelong exposure to estrogens, the higher her risk of breast cancer; the higher a woman's aromatase level in tissues, the greater her estrogen levels will be; the greater her percent of body fat, the higher her aromatase activity. Unequivocally we can say that keeping the body weight as low as possible without being underweight is a good strategy for reducing risk of post-menopausal breast cancer.

Parenthetically, you may also want to know what else increases aromatase levels so you can reduce it in other ways. One factor that increases aromatase is simply the process of getting older, a risk factor we can't do anything about, regardless of the extravagant claims of the "anti-aging" doctors.

Alcohol intake also increases aromatase activity, which may be one reason that alcohol intake at any level seems to increase risk of breast cancer. And by the way, breast cancer is not the only malignancy that becomes more likely with alcohol intake. It is safe to say that alcohol is an overall cancer promoter, at least when intake is immoderate. Low to moderate alcohol intake seems to have some health benefits.

This is a complex topic that I will explore in more detail later, but for now, you just need to know that alcohol, even at moderate levels of intake, increases risk of breast cancer.

Before—or After—Menopause?

On the other hand, when looking at risk factors for premenopausal breast cancer, excess weight seems to be a protective factor. Women who are overweight are less likely than normal-weight women to develop breast cancer before menopause. Since being overweight has a protective benefit, does it make sense to purposely keep or acquire excess weight before menopause? The answer is clearly no, for several reasons.

One reason to avoid excess weight before menopause is that most women who are overweight before menopause will continue to be overweight after menopause. I do not need to remind anyone of the number of women who remain frustrated at their ineffective efforts to drop those extra pounds when they would like to. Another reason is that excess weight at any age increases disease risk in so many other ways; most notably is the risk of cardiovascular disease, Type 2 diabetes and other forms of cancer.

Because premenopausal breast cancer is a much rarer disease than postmenopausal breast cancer, the absolute numbers of women who would be protected by that added weight is relatively small. There would, however, be a much larger number of women who would be at risk of cancer because of the obesity that they carried from their premenopausal to postmenopausal years.

If for no other reason than to set the record straight, I want you to know that being overweight is a protective factor against premenopausal breast cancer. However, I do not believe this has any practical implications as a health strategy. This will prove to be useful information only if in the future we clarify why this is protective, and then are able to isolate the step that translates that protection and confer it to women without the extra weight. I have little doubt that in the near future, advances in research will make that possible. In the meantime, aim for a lean body mass.

How Exercise Prevents Cancer

And on that note, now is a perfect opportunity to talk about exercise and its cancer-preventing potential. Over 25 years of medical practice, I have been consulted by countless patients wanting my advice on how to most effectively get rid of the extra pounds they are carrying. I am more convinced than ever that daily physical activity is the critical foundational step for that, whether for adolescents or for the elderly. Exercise builds muscle, and even if the weight stays the same, a pound of muscle burns more energy than a pound of fat, even while you are sleeping.

A body that has a higher proportion of muscle mass is also less likely to display a phenomenon called insulin resistance. Practically speaking, this means that a person with better-developed and toned muscles requires the pancreas to put out proportionately less insulin to maintain normal blood sugar. And a person with poorly developed muscles and a large percentage of body fat will display insulin resistance, meaning that the tissues will need higher and higher levels of insulin in order to maintain a normal level of blood sugar. This puts a strain on the pancreas, which eventually cannot keep up with the demand for greater levels of insulin—and diabetes inevitably develops.

For the purpose of this discussion on cancer prevention, it is important to understand the way insulin works in the body beyond its role in blood sugar control.

Insulin is a growth promoter of body tissues in general, a hormone that doctors describe as "anabolic." Insulin is the most powerful hormone in the body that makes cells and tissues grow. On the deficiency side, this is why when insulin becomes deficient (in Type 1, or *juvenile diabetes*), an untreated individual will lose weight uncontrollably, and, before artificial insulin became available for injection, those Type 1 diabetes patients would always die soon after developing the disease.

However, when insulin is in excess, in response to an overweight body that is resistant to its action, it promotes growth of body tissues in a sometimes unhealthy way. For example, insulin promotes the growth of tumors. This is why people with Type 2 diabetes have higher rates of cancer than the general population.

But here is the good news: you can do something about it.

Starting today, starting now, you can begin a habit of moving your body in healthy and enjoyable ways, to build muscle, to burn calories, to make healthy weight control possible.

If you have arthritis, chronic pain or any sort of disability, ask your doctor for a referral to a physical therapist to help devise an exercise program that is realistic for you. Often beginning in a warm water therapy pool or in water aerobics is a great way to start if you are physically challenged.

If you have heart disease or perhaps are not sure if you might, ask your doctor about the advisability of getting a cardiac evaluation (stress test) before starting an exercise program.

And please, if you have not been accustomed to daily exercise, start slowly. Give yourself a schedule of small realistic goals, and find a success partner who will either exercise with you or who will have your permission to call you regularly to celebrate your successes and encourage you when you feel you are not keeping up.

Maybe now would be a good time to put this book down, and go for a walk!

Put to Rest the Contrary Rumors

Parenthetically, I need to add that even though a very few studies have associated the highest levels of exercise with increased risk of breast cancer (and of course this made headlines), the preponderance of medical evidence and expert opinion is strongly in favor of exercise (even the highest levels of exercise) as being protective. Those negative studies are the exception, not the rule. To support that position, a study published in 2007 looked at California teachers, and found that strenuous physical activity for at least five hours a week was protective against breast cancer compared to women in the lowest activity level.[1]

Clearly the weight of evidence is in favor of exercise as a protective strategy against breast cancer, and if you are a competitive athlete, you do not have to worry about such activity increasing your risk. Not only is exercise protective against its development, regular exercise in women who have already been diagnosed with breast cancer is associated with improved rates of survival. This is true for vigorous exercise and also true for gentle exercises like Qigong (chee-kung) and yoga.

We are talking about exercise, and this necessarily brings up thoughts of breast support and sports bras. It would be an excellent time to put to rest rumors that brassieres are a risk factor for breast cancer. This has been discussed in some popular books and circulated on the Internet, but I can find no convincing evidence that this is true, and other expert bodies (such as the American Cancer Society) agree. Feel free to enjoy wearing a bra that provides support during exercise and daily life if that is your preference, without fear that it is harmful.

Other Fabulous Benefits of Exercise

As I said in the introduction, one of the reasons I am so confident in making the recommendations in this book is that their risks are low to nonexistent. And their benefits extend far beyond cancer prevention, whether we are talking about food choices or physical activity. Making some physical activity a part of your daily routine is a foundation for health throughout your lifespan. Besides reduction of cancer risk, other benefits of exercise include the following:

- Improved bone health: regular physical activity is the single most important determinant of good bone density in women, preventing osteoporosis.
- Improved mood: exercise has been measured as an intervention in depression and works as well as some prescription anti-depressants.
- Reduced risk of cardiovascular disease: physical inactivity (a sedentary lifestyle) doubles one's risk of dying of heart disease![2]
- Reducing weight and obesity: people who remain physically active on a regular basis are more likely to be close to their ideal body weight. Reduction in obesity of course has medical benefits, but on a day-to-day basis, the positive emotional impact of feeling good about one's size and shape is at least as important to many, if not most, women.

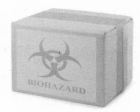

CHAPTER 3
Minimizing Environmental Toxins

When I was a young teenager, my grandfather was diagnosed with colon cancer. I still have a vivid memory of my father sitting down at the family dinner table and announcing to all of his children, "J.B. has cancer."

My grandfather Pendergrast was known all of his life by his initials, J.B. He was a pharmacist and owned his own drugstore in Atlanta during the rapid growth of that city from the early to the latter half of the 20th century. From the time he took his first job until retirement, he worked seven days a week. In those early years, pharmacists compounded medicines in their own stores and could prescribe for their customers based on symptoms. He would not recognize the regulations of today.

By the late 1960s, when the malignancy was growing in his colon, he had slowed down and had been able to enjoy some of the fruits of a life of hard work and thrift. He did not survive long after that diagnosis. There was not much to do for metastatic colon cancer in an elderly man around 1970. My final memory of that chapter in my family's life was at the graveside, seeing my grandmother barely able to see where she was stepping for all the tears in her eyes.

Even at that young age, long before I was to study medicine, I wondered what caused that cancer. I had heard that smoking caused lung cancer, so I assumed there must be some analogous toxin for the colon. Was it something he ate or smoked—a toxic compound to which he was exposed in the pharmacy? Research for the past 40 years has shed a lot of light on just those questions.

How Does Cancer Start?

What happens to a perfectly normal cell, functioning as it should, to shift its "mission" from one of teamwork to unbridled growth at the expense of all other tissue; uncontrolled growth eventually leading to the death of the host unless checked and stopped? And why would one person be more likely to be diagnosed with cancer than a near neighbor, relative or family member?

There is no question that genetics plays a role in answering those questions, and massive amounts of research and money are being poured into unlocking the genetic predispositions to various cancers so that we will know better how to prevent them. But at the time of this writing, your genetic inheritance is at best something to be aware of, but not something you can modify. Your genes are your genes, for now at least. (Although I expect in the near future that medical technology will evolve to the point of being able to address and modify even genetic risk).

Genetic risk is a real but unwavering factor in "why" cancers start, but the major risk that is modifiable is the presence of environmental toxins. In this brief overview, the following toxins will be explored:

- Ionizing radiation,
- Chemical carcinogens,
- Xenoestrogens (compounds that mimic the action of natural body hormones),
- Hormones in our meat and dairy supply, and finally,
- The effect of environmental changes like habitual sleep patterns and exposure to light.

Radiation as a Carcinogen

The word carcinogen means, very simply, a compound or energy that can initiate the growth of cancer where there was none. The possibility that environmental toxins may initiate the process of cancer has been known since the early 20th century.

Historically, the tragic story of Marie Curie is illustrative. Curie, a brilliant scientist and winner of two Nobel prizes, devoted her career to unlocking the mysteries of radiation. She herself realized very quickly that these discoveries would form the basis for technologies useful in medicine, both as diagnostic X-rays and as radiation treatments for cancer. But she was not aware that prolonged exposure to the same radiation would unalterably modify the genetics of her blood cell precursors in the bone marrow, and she eventually died of aplastic anemia, a failure of the bone marrow to make new blood.

Certainly on a more massively tragic scale, the greatest radiation exposures to human populations of the 20th century have been the nuclear weapons dropped on Japanese citizens during World War II, and the Chernobyl nuclear reactor explosion in 1986 that released much more radiation into the environment than both the nuclear bombs combined. In the 10 years following the Chernobyl disaster it is estimated that in Europe 1000 new cases of thyroid cancer and 4000 cases of other cancers were due to the radiation release into the environment.[1]

The health consequences for those who survived the immediate effects have been an increased risk of cancer at almost every body site. And risk continues for decades after the initial exposure. This is the reason that hospital employees and doctors who work in radiology departments must wear protective clothing and also carry radiation exposure detectors on their person every minute at work; keeping track of cumulative exposure to radiation allows the conscious choice to limit that exposure to known, safer levels.

X-rays are one form of a general category called *ionizing radiation.* Other forms of ionizing radiation that are commonly present in our environments are UV rays (from the sun) and cosmic rays from space (which are more common in the upper atmosphere than at the earth's surface). Any form of ionizing radiation is capable of initiating the growth of cancer without any other risk factors being present.

Sunlight, Vitamin D, and Breast Health

With regard to breast cancer, sun exposure (despite the UV rays) is a good thing and a preventive strategy because the skin converts other steroid compounds in the skin to vitamin D on exposure to sunlight. Evidence suggests that vitamin D may play a role in prevention of breast cancer. In summer it only takes 15 minutes of mid-day sun on your skin (in swimsuit or shorts) to produce your daily vitamin D requirement or more.

Mammograms and Radiation Exposure

X-ray exposure of the breasts brings up more problematic questions. While current diagnostic X-ray technology is designed to minimize radiation exposure to any single individual, there is no "floor" below which one can say, "This dose of radiation to your breast tissue carries no risk." In fact, any radiation dose increases risk of cancer, no matter how miniscule that increase may be.

My response to that as a doctor is to think twice before I order a chest X-ray, and ask myself if this is really necessary for the best care of my patient. Sometimes I believe it is, and we proceed with an X-ray.

There are some who object to this diagnostic screening using mammograms for that very reason. And it is awareness of this reality that has pushed the evolution of mammogram technology to require less and less radiation exposure over the last 20 years or so. Recognizing that even the very low dose of radiation required to perform a mammogram increases risk of cancer even a tiny amount, I am hopeful that new technologies that are under research will make the mammogram obsolete in the future.

For the present, though, the mammogram is still a useful tool that saves lives by early detection of breast cancer in an early, curable stage. If you are over 40, please follow current guidelines for mammogram screening.[2]

How Does a Carcinogen Work?

Understanding the process of what happens to a cell when exposed to a carcinogen is perhaps easiest understood in the context of radiation and cells, but the principles are applicable to chemical carcinogens as well. Please understand that this is an enormous simplification of a very complex topic. To begin, all human cells contain DNA, the *blueprint* for how the cell is to function.

The role of the DNA is to produce RNA, which then produces proteins that regulate cell function. Part of that cell instruction manual, written in proteins, is to tell the cell how often to divide and create offspring cells, when to stop dividing, and when to die when its work is done. If the DNA is damaged quite severely, the cell will simply die. It was such massive cell death from high dose radiation exposure that killed so many people in the days and weeks following Hiroshima, Nagasaki and Chernobyl.

When DNA is damaged by a lower dose of radiation—a non-lethal dose—a mutation occurs. The accumulation of mutations over time may eventually produce a line of cells that has lost its boundaries and does not follow the original DNA rules about how often to divide, when to stop dividing and when to die. Any one cell with non-lethal DNA damage can divide, producing copies of itself that have no instructions on stopping division or dying, and this is the beginning of cancer.

Non-lethal DNA damage may occur as the result of exposure to any number of environmental carcinogens. For the most part, a higher dose and a longer period of time of exposure increase the likelihood that the cancerous transformation will occur.

Chemicals Which Cause Cancer

What are some known chemical carcinogens to avoid or to which one should minimize exposure? My short list here will not include some of the most toxic carcinogens, because many of those are uncommon enough in the environment that you are not likely to be exposed in a significant way. The ones I choose to highlight here are those to which you may be exposed in the course of everyday life, and about which you can do something to minimize risk.

Stay Away from These

Tobacco smoke has been a known carcinogen for decades now. Doctors and the public first became aware of this association with regard to lung cancer and its increase within the general population. The effects of inhaled tobacco smoke (whether by the smoker or by those in the nearby environment of the smoker, i.e. secondhand smoke) extend far beyond just lung cancer. A 2006 review of 40 years of research data from Japan revealed a significant number of studies in which tobacco smoke increased the risk of breast cancer. Not all studies showed the association, but it certainly lends a note of extreme caution to a very plausible and modifiable contributor to breast cancer risk.[3]

Polychlorinated biphenyls (PCBs) are industrial chemicals that have been widely used in plastics, paints and adhesives. These do not break down easily in the environment. As a result, they can enter the food chain and are then stored in the fat tissue of animals. The presence of PCBs is a known risk factor for breast cancer. Avoiding or at least limiting consumption of PCBs can be accomplished by being aware of their sources in our food supply and making wise choices.

> **One of the easiest is to know which fish are likely to be contaminated with PCBs, and choosing other healthy fish.[4] Farm-raised salmon is currently one of the fish types known to be an unsafe source of PCBs, and I suggest avoiding those fish and consuming only wild salmon instead.**

Another common cancer-causing chemical exposure is the presence of heterocyclic amines and polycyclic aromatic hydrocarbons formed from cooking meat at high temperatures. This is especially true of grilling meat, chicken or fish if it results in any charring. Charred meat does (not *maybe*; it *does*) contain polycyclic aromatic hydrocarbons when it comes off the grill. Even if not charred, it seems likely that the longer a meat is exposed to very high temperatures, the more likely it will be a significant source of carcinogens.

A study supporting this assertion showed that women who stated a preference to eat their beef "well done" were more likely to later report breast cancer. In fact, consumption of well done, fried or barbecued meat is now known to be a breast cancer risk.[5]

It is also known that the addition of nitrates or nitrites to meats as a preservative (such as in processed deli meats) can lead to cancer, because these form N-nitroso compounds (some of which are known carcinogens) in the meat or in the individual consuming the preservative-rich meat. My advice on meat: eat less, and when you do eat it, avoid meat with preservatives such as nitrates, and enjoy your steak cooked medium at most. Slow cooking at lower heat would seem to be a better choice judging from the data.

The addition of chlorine to the drinking water supply in many industrialized nations has led to dramatic decreases in water-borne infections. Safe drinking water is still a major public health concern around the world, and chlorination has helped to create clean water in many parts of the world.

However, from what we know now about the health effects of chlorine in our tap water, it is time for new technology to take over the job of disinfecting the water supply. Chlorine is a very toxic gas, and it reacts very easily with organic compounds present in municipal water supplies to form a class of chemicals called trihalomethanes, or THMs. The presence of THMs in the drinking water supply is now known to be a risk factor for cancers of the bladder and colon/rectum.[6] While there are some data linking THM and chlorine exposure to breast cancer development, those data are not as conclusive as the bladder and colon research.

> While the research is unfolding, why expose yourself knowingly to a carcinogen? I urge you to get a filter for your drinking water at home, and also to install a filter on your shower head and bathtub if possible, because breathing the chlorine and its byproducts is just as dangerous, if not more so, than drinking it.

Chemicals that Mimic Estrogen

Pesticides and plastics also deserve some discussion and your attention. With regard to breast cancer, the pertinent problem is that many chemical pesticides used in farms and gardens act as xenoestrogens. A xenoestrogen is a compound that has no *natural place* in human life, but which by chance (very bad luck) interacts with human tissue and triggers a response that would normally be reserved for a human hormone.

Pesticides act as xenoestrogens when they bind to estrogen receptors in the body (specifically the breast) and cause those receptors to become active as if there were higher levels of estrogen circulating. That artificial chemical stimulating estrogen receptors could promote the growth of estrogen sensitive tumors.

Similar compounds also enter the body through exposure to some plastics, such as when foods placed in a plastic container are heated in a microwave oven and the plastic compounds that act like estrogens leach into the food. As you might have guessed by now, I am suggesting that you minimize xenoestrogen exposure by choosing organically grown produce whenever possible and by not cooking or storing food (or water) in plastic containers.[7]

Just Say No to Hormones in Your Food

The role of hormones used in dairy and meat production also deserves a cautionary note. The treatment of dairy cows with rBGH (recombinant bovine growth hormone) is a controversial topic. (It is also called rBST—recombinant bovine somatotropin). While I know of no studies linking such milk to human cancers, breast or otherwise, I believe there is reason for caution and avoidance until we prove (if ever) that there is not a problem here. We know that the rBGH/rBST is not actively excreted in the cow's milk, so you as the consumer are not put at risk by the rBGH/rBST itself. But that same milk does have higher levels of another hormone in it called insulin-like growth factor, or IGF-1.

Good science has shown that IGF-1 is a tumor growth promoter; in other words, that set of mutated cells growing out of control tends to multiply faster in the presence of IGF-1. I believe this is reason enough to insist on consuming only dairy products that have not come from cows treated with rBGH/rBST.

> **Read the labels in the store: if it does not say "certified organic" or "rBGH/rBST free," there is a very good chance those cows were exposed and that milk is unsafe in my opinion.**

Similar concerns exist about beef, because much of the conventionally raised beef consumed in this country comes from cows that are treated regularly with growth hormones to add weight and size. Residual growth hormones may be present in that meat in sufficient quantities to also act as tumor promoters in humans, similar to the milk concern. The science on this topic is not conclusive about any increased cancer risk. However, I still believe the precautionary principle applies: Do not knowingly expose yourself to a substance about which there is reasonable concern when you have an alternative. Decrease meat consumption, and choose grass-fed, non-hormone-treated beef.

Melatonin and Sleep

One final environmental note has to do with one's working environment, and how it impacts sleep. Research has found that women who consistently work a night shift have higher rates of breast cancer. It is theorized that melatonin, the natural hormone our bodies make during sleep and darkness, is decreased in these women over time, and that melatonin has a protective role against breast cancer.

If you have compelling reasons to work a night shift, I would not let this concern stop you; but I would suggest an extra dose of caution in minimizing other known risk factors. If you have the opportunity to change to working mostly daylight hours and sleeping at night, that would seem to be a healthy decision.

PART 2

Top 10 Foods for
Breast Health

Here in Part 2, we will review together 10 real foods that I believe can be among your strongest allies in maintaining health and reducing your risk of breast cancer. But . . .

*If you have turned to this page by skipping Part 1,
please stop and go back.*

The principles laid out in the Introduction and Part 1 are foundational to your understanding of cancer prevention strategies. This section focuses on single foods that are powerful friends of yours. However, no single food is as important as the varied diet and lifestyle principles that are discussed in Part 1.

Thanks for being patient with the book and the process by which I am trying to empower you step-by-step to stay healthy. I am purposely keeping these chapters short. Every woman wants to reduce her cancer risk. I believe you want practical information and recommendations for the foods you can choose to reduce that risk, not a long scientific review of research articles. Read on; the answers are in your hands.

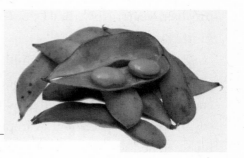

CHAPTER 4
The Joy of Soy—
and Some Cautions

S oy foods are one of the most important foods we know about for breast cancer prevention. It's a great addition to our diets and has proven health benefits, but it is not as simple as standing on a street corner holding a sign up to all passersby saying,

Eat More Soy.

There are some products made from soybeans or edible extracts of soybeans that I do not believe you should be eating. The science on how soy foods may protect against breast cancer also indicates that a woman's age has a great deal to do with how well this strategy works. For some women, specifically those with estrogen-receptor positive breast cancer already, there is quite a bit of controversy on soy recommendations. My current reading of the science is that it is too early to draw any conclusions (more on this topic in a few moments).

My wife and I introduced soy into our children's diets at young ages. We used firm tofu in stir-fries, used edamame as a cooked vegetable, and even "spiked" smoothies for the unsuspecting with a little soft tofu. When my youngest daughter was a toddler, tofu was one of her favorite foods. She could not get enough of it and would demand more when her serving was gone. I did not know the data then about the impact of soy on cancer prevention, especially in girls during childhood and pre-teen years. Now that I do, I am glad she had those foods early in life.

More recently, when my children became teenagers, they became more suspicious of "healthy" foods in general. And if I was the one cooking for dinner, they had good reason to be suspicious. I still "hide" soy in recipes, especially if I can put it in the blender for sauces, or use unsweetened soy milk as a dairy substitute when baking, or using part soy flour in place of part of the wheat flour.

If the spaghetti sauce was a little different color than one might expect, you would hear at the table, "Dad, did you put tofu in this?" My reading on the topic convinces me it is worth the reaction; the benefits are clear, despite some controversy—and their reactions.

Few topics in the science of food's influence on cancer risk have provoked more controversy lately, so it's good to take this one out for some sunshine early in our journey together. It's a good time to re-emphasize some fundamental principles of what we know about using foods for cancer risk reduction. They apply especially to soy foods.

Reducing cancer risk through food choices has to do more with the variety and combinations of foods in the diet than one single food. There is no single magic food that you can concentrate on to the exclusion of a balance. It's better to get your cancer risk reduction from whole foods than from pills, concentrates or supplements. And, there is no 100 percent guaranteed way to prevent cancers by food choices; the goal is to move yourself into a lower risk group.

Soy and Breast Cancer Prevention

Here's what we know about soy foods. Higher intake of soy foods in a population (such as women in countries of eastern Asia) is associated with lower rates of breast cancer in those countries. This is a consistent finding in research studies of large populations of women, whether in their home countries in Asia, or Asian immigrants to the U.S. whose dietary patterns differ from other American women.[1] A 2006 review of a large number of studies of Japanese and Chinese women showed specifically that women who consumed tofu and other soy foods in their diets had lower rates of breast cancer.[2]

Researchers suggest that the protective effects of soy on the breast come from its phytoestrogen properties (its ability to partly block estrogen receptors in the breast), and is related to high concentrations of a class of compounds called isoflavones. Isoflavones are a specific subtype of flavonoids. Flavonoids are widely distributed in vegetable foods, and all of the studies ever done on flavonoids support their cancer protective properties.

Like other legumes, soy is high in folate, phytic acid and oligosaccharides (prebiotics that promote growth of healthy bacteria and promote colon health), all of which have anticancer properties; these legumes also protect against heart disease, and diabetes, and help to promote bone health. Soy for men also has been shown to be protective against prostate cancer.

The strongest evidence for the role of soy foods in breast cancer prevention is actually in premenopausal women, rather than in preventing post-menopausal breast cancer (the more common variety). This has been speculatively thought to be due to the combined properties of soy isoflavones as both estrogenic and anti-estrogenic at the same time.

It is thought that soy isoflavones exert an antiestrogenic effect in a high estrogen environment (premenopausal women), and a very weak estrogenic effect in a low-estrogen environment (post-menopausal women and in men). This aligns nicely with laboratory data from animal studies showing that soy is most likely to have a protective effect against breast cancer if consumed while the breast is still developing, as in pre-teen and adolescent girls.

My reading of the science at this time is that we have enough data to conclude that soy can protect against breast cancer by reducing the total estrogenic stimulation of the breast during premenopausal years, especially in young girls. The data supporting the role of soy in preventing post-menopausal breast cancer is more limited and speculative. The circumstantial evidence for protecting against post-menopausal breast cancer is reasonably defensible in my opinion. Not from consuming soy in the post-menopausal years, but because soy consumption in childhood, adolescence and young adulthood can lower the cumulative estrogen stimulation of the breast over a lifetime. We do know that the duration of high estrogen levels in a woman's body is a definite risk factor for post-menopausal breast cancer.

Soy Foods if You Already Have Breast Cancer

The studies on soy's effect on women who already have breast cancer is conflicting, some showing a harmful effect, and some showing that higher isoflavone intake increases survival rates in breast cancer patients. There have been some concerns that soy foods (isoflavones) could interfere with tamoxifen during cancer treatment. But in support of soy foods, the most recent data from 2009 found that women on tamoxifen for cancer treatment who consumed the highest levels of soy proteins actually greatly reduced their risk of recurrence and the soy did not interfere with tamoxifen efficacy.[3] Sound confusing? Here's my conclusion:

Soy is a good food choice, and should especially be encouraged for school-age and teenage girls. Adult women can enjoy soy foods, especially if it is one of your legume choices to replace meat as a protein source. It is not clear yet from studies whether we can endorse soy foods as protective for women who already have breast cancer or whether there are any women for whom soy could interfere with treatment.

What we can say at this time is, "The best science has not given clear direction on this point."

I only recommend getting soy from whole foods and *not* from soy isoflavone concentrates in pills, and *not* from soy protein powders as are often found in instant breakfast drink powders or "meat substitute" products in which textured soy protein (highly processed soy) is used to make a food that looks like meat but is not.

Some Real Soy Foods to Enjoy

Edamame is a great place to start if you are new to soy foods. It is the whole soy bean, boiled and either in the shell (like peas in a pod) or out of it (in which case it looks sort of like a round green lima bean). You will find it served alongside sushi in Japanese restaurants. You can buy it in the frozen food section of the grocery and either heat and serve as an appetizer or snack alone, or put it liberally on your salad with other vegetables of various colors.

Tofu is another good choice as a whole soy food. Because of the way tofu is made (curdled soy milk) using calcium salts, it is an excellent source of calcium in addition to the benefits already noted. I recommend only non-GMO, organically grown soy.

Be aware also that some of the soy milk beverages on the market are high enough in sugar as to concern me for their high glycemic index. Though it may take some time, I think you can become accustomed to using the unsweetened soy beverages on your morning breakfast cereal. I also caution people to watch out for beverages that have been "smoothed out" by using carrageenan, a ubiquitous additive in the American food market, sometimes found on food labels as "Irish moss." There are actually very few soy beverages in the grocery stores that do not have carrageenan added for texture. (Mouth feel is a very important marketing concept for food companies, evidently because it is so important to American buyers.)

Carrageenan is still on the FDA's "generally recognized as safe" list, but there are laboratory studies which make me doubt if that is appropriate. It has been commonly used in animal studies to experimentally induce colitis in lab animals so that researchers can study new potential treatments for inflammatory bowel diseases like Crohn's and ulcerative colitis.

Here's the bottom line on soy: Enjoy whole soy foods such as edamame, tofu, miso and soy beverages (preferably unsweetened and without carrageenan), and, for members of your family, the younger the better (even during infancy there is no convincing evidence for harm of soy based formula, but breast feeding is always best). Soy food consumption has many health benefits in addition to its cancer protective role, and when you share with the significant men in your life, they too will reap the health benefits.

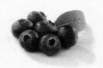

CHAPTER 5
Cruciferous Vegetables

Here's a quick trivia quiz question: Which modern U.S. president became famous for his dislike of broccoli? I'll let you stew over that question for a while, and before we reveal the answer, you will have many reasons to feel sorry for the poor man!

The family of cruciferous vegetables has special significance when it comes to cancer prevention, especially breast cancer prevention. This family includes some familiar and some less familiar vegetable names: broccoli, cauliflower, cabbage, brussel sprouts, kale, turnips, mustard greens and bok choy, among others. They are known by their botanical family name, the *Brassica* vegetables.

Cruciferous vegetables got their name because their flowers have four petals in a cross-like shape (a crucifer). While I am continuing to recommend that you enjoy a wide variety of vegetables and fruits daily for maximum health benefit, this particular family of vegetables deserves special attention because of some natural compounds that are uniquely concentrated in these edible powerhouses.

Vegetables in the *Brassica* family are rich sources of compounds called isothiocyanates and indoles (don't worry; there will not be a quiz or a spelling bee). Specific and prominent examples of these are sulforaphane and indole-3-carbinol (I3C), both of which have been found in research to have potent anticancer properties. With regard to breast cancer prevention, it is worth discussing I3C in more detail. In studies where women have been supplemented with I3C, the body shows biochemical signs of shifting the metabolism of estrogen away from a 16 hydroxyl form to a 2 hydroxyl form.

Why would you care? Simply this: The 2 hydroxyl is your friend. When the 16 hydroxyl form of estrogen is most active in the body, it is more likely to promote tumor growth than the less active 2 hydroxyl form. And when I3C is present, a larger portion of estrogen is metabolized in the liver to the 2 hydroxyl form, which is relatively inactive. In theory it would not be as likely to promote tumor growth.

> **The longer a woman is exposed to estrogen over her lifetime, the higher her breast cancer risk.**

Laboratory studies in animal models have shown a decreased number of breast tumors when I3C is in the diet, probably because of the favorable 2 hydroxyl form being more dominant. Interestingly, and importantly, recent research in cell cultures in laboratories has shown that I3C also inhibits growth and metastasis of existing breast cancer cells.

In addition to the role of I3C in shifting estrogen to a less active form that may be less likely to promote tumor growth, the cruciferous vegetables play an important role in helping the liver do its job of protecting the body against environmental toxins. Because high levels of indoles and isothiocyanates promote the activity of the natural enzymes that work in the liver to detoxify our systems, cabbage and its relatives also are able to promote detoxification of potentially dangerous compounds when they reach the liver. They thus help to minimize the cancer-causing risk of environmental pollutants.

All of the information above is based on laboratory studies, and it is very promising in terms of the role of cruciferous vegetables in reducing cancer risk. But does it play out in real life? Again there is evidence for this in large studies of women in different population groups.

For example, a study of women from Long Island, published in 2007, showed that women with the highest dietary intake of flavones had an almost 40 percent lower risk of breast cancer.[1] It is known that cruciferous vegetables are especially good vegetable sources of this class of phytonutrients called flavones. This is consistent with other previous research, which showed that higher intake of any type of flavonoid nutrient protected women against breast cancer. Be sure to expand their intake in your diet.

Whole Foods vs. Supplements

These studies of real women in real life bring up an important point. The data we have on people (not laboratory experiments) that support the consumption of cruciferous vegetables for cancer prevention are from the consumption of the whole foods, not supplements in pill form. While it is possible to buy dietary supplements and take quite high doses of I3C or other compounds found in these foods, we have no long-term data saying that this is either a safe or effective strategy for cancer prevention. For both safety and efficacy, I would prefer, and highly recommend, that you get your phytonutrients from whole foods, not from dietary supplements.

Cabbage, Broccoli and Cauliflower

In addition to all the reliable scientific information I can provide, I also have a goal of giving you the confidence that you can find ways to enjoy these lifesaving foods even if you have not enjoyed them in the past. Personally, I have liked cabbage as long as I can remember. And, I confess, steamed cabbage with a little salt and pepper is one of my comfort foods.

Unfortunately, cabbage has been portrayed in literature and in the cinema as being the boring food of choice for poor people. That's the myth I'd like to dispel right now. Cabbage is anything but boring (and there are much more interesting ways to cook it than steaming)! And the most interesting of all the cabbages I have met is the red/purple variety.

Even before we get to its anticancer properties, red cabbage is a healthy food in many ways. It is an excellent source of fiber, vitamin C, vitamin K and vitamin A (as natural carotenoids such as beta carotene, lutein and zeaxanthin). It is very low in fats of course, and of the tiny amount of natural fats that do occur in this lovely vegetable, omega 3 fatty acids are one of the largest components. It also has a very low glycemic index, meaning it does not raise blood sugar in an unhealthy way.

Red cabbage is one of the great foods for specifically reducing risk of breast cancer, for several reasons. The pigment that makes red cabbage red is called an anthocyanin, which is a type of flavonoid. Flavonoids have been extensively studied, and women whose diets are higher in flavonoids have a reduced risk of breast cancer. I recommend that you cook this vegetable in order to release the highest levels of antioxidants; a stir-fry in olive oil with some other chopped vegetables, onion and garlic would be not only healing but also delicious and interesting!

Broccoli in the past 30 years has made a move from the back of the pack to near "front runner" status in vegetable popularity rankings. Americans' favorite vegetables are still white potatoes (my advice is to minimize those) and tomatoes (good stuff), but broccoli consumption in the U.S. has increased more than 160 percent since the 1970s, according to the USDA. And except for the "anti-broccoli gang" (like our former president), that's really good news for health. The other good news is that broccoli is not even in the top 20 most pesticide-laden foods in your produce section, so conventionally grown is still a relatively safe choice (even though I support organic agriculture for all crops).

In addition to its cancer-preventing properties, broccoli is a healthy food in many ways. It is an excellent source of fiber, vitamin A (as natural carotenoids), vitamin C (one large stalk will provide more than 300 percent of your daily vitamin C needs!), vitamin E (natural tocopherols), vitamin K, the B vitamins and potassium. It also has a very low glycemic index. And you may be surprised to know that a single serving of broccoli can provide more than 300 milligrams of omega-3 fatty acids, adding to its anti-inflammatory properties. All of these qualities also make it a front-runner for preventing heart disease as well.

And who was the anti-broccoli president? George Bush, Sr. of course, who apparently felt so obliged to clean his plate for his mother that it took becoming "leader of the free world" for him to declare his vegetable independence: "I do not like broccoli. And I haven't liked it since I was a little kid and my mother made me eat it. And I'm President of the United States and I'm not going to eat any more broccoli." Too bad, Mr. President. I hope you've been taking your vitamins.

Cauliflower is next on my list for some special emphasis. I am also relieved to be finally writing about a vegetable that is white, but good for you (in general I will advise you to avoid white foods, e.g. white rice, potatoes and much bread, because of their glycemic index). As children, my siblings and I were prompted by its ghostly white color to derisively call cauliflower "dead broccoli." But as you will see by its nutritional content, it is anything but dead.

Cauliflower is full of powerful health benefits even before enumerating its anticancer properties. It is an excellent source of fiber, and a half-cup of cooked cauliflower provides more than 25 milligrams of vitamin C, a moderate amount of folate, and even though it is a very low-fat food, that same serving gives you more than 100 milligrams of healthy omega-3 fatty acids. And like broccoli, it also has a very low glycemic index.

Those are just a few of the examples of the specific members of the cruciferous family (Brassica) of vegetables, and how they are not only a great cancer prevention strategy, but also can be enjoyed in a variety of ways every day.

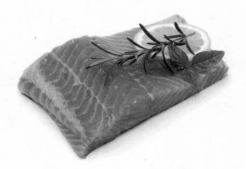

CHAPTER 6
Go Fish

You can hardly pick up a health-related magazine these days without finding something about the health benefits of fish, especially those "oily" cold-water fish like salmon and sardines. Being a well-informed and health-conscious eater, you certainly are aware now that increasing our dietary intake of omega-3 fatty acids is an essential health strategy. The typical American diet has a very high omega-6 to omega-3 ratio, and bringing that ratio lower will reduce the risk of many chronic diseases.

You can do that by decreasing your use of vegetable cooking oils (corn oil, safflower oil, peanut oil and soy oils, especially those used in baked goods) and increasing intake of oily cold-water fish (for non-fish eaters, we will talk later about vegetarian options for increasing omega-3 fats).

Fish Oils: a Foundation of Preventive Medicine

This one strategy is such a key to good health that I find it to be a foundation of my medical recommendations in almost all of my Integrative Medicine consults at my office, for adults and children alike. The scientific literature is full of studies showing that higher levels of these healthy fats is associated with lower rates of chronic diseases such as rheumatoid arthritis, heart disease, ulcerative colitis and even psoriasis. Fish oils (and their active component, the omega-3 fats) have been associated with increased HDL (good) cholesterol, lowered triglyceride levels, decreased risk of fatal heart rhythm problems in people after a heart attack, decreased risk of sudden death in people with *no* history of heart disease, improvements in depression, and slower progression of degenerative brain diseases. They have a modest tendency to make blood platelets less sticky, so clots are less likely. This could in theory pose a risk to someone who is already taking blood thinners, so if that is your situation, discuss the advisability of fish oil with your doctor (though I have personally not seen that to be a problem).

With the huge positive potential and the minimal downside, should we all be taking fish oil? One could make a case for that unless you happen to eat at least two six-ounce servings of cold-water oily fish per week already.

> **Solid science also links higher levels of these omega-3 oils to reduced risk of cancers, including colon, prostate and breast cancer.**

How Do Fish Oils Decrease Cancer Risk?

An extremely technical paper in *Biomedicine & Pharmacotherapy* (2002) reviewed the chemistry and how the active components in fish oil work in your body.[1] A class of enzymes called cyclo-oxygenases (COX for short) is involved in producing inflammatory compounds in the body called prostaglandins. There are two types of COX: COX-1 and COX-2. COX-2 is the one most involved in pain and inflammation, but it also creates a tissue environment that promotes tumor growth. High levels of COX-2 activity are found in breast and colon tumors. And DHA (that good fat found in fish) down-regulates the activity of COX-2 in tissues.

Additionally, there are many experimental and laboratory studies that show that omega-3 fatty acids inhibit the growth of breast tumors. But the results of large-scale population studies have been mixed; some showing that fish or fish oil intake reduces breast cancer risk, and some showing no association with risk. More importantly, none has shown that fish increases risk of cancer.

Two recent studies from Asia, published in 2007, shed more light on the topic. Researchers measured omega-3 and other fatty acid levels in the blood cells of women with and without breast cancer and compared the levels. The much higher omega-3 levels in the blood of women without breast cancer in both studies suggest again that fish or fish oil intake could be protective against disease. My conclusion is that the evidence points overwhelmingly to an important role for oily fish consumption in the prevention of cancer, both from population studies and from the laboratory.

My Recommendation?

> **Women should be eating cold-water fish twice weekly, and possibly taking a fish oil supplement, to reduce breast cancer risk.**

Those fish meals should replace some intake of red meat and other saturated fats in the diet, since saturated fats (we get those mostly from meats and dairy) are associated with more inflammation in the body. I acknowledge the scientific purists who would say the data are conflicting on the topic, but I believe their insistence on stronger evidence is not needed here because of the well-known other benefits of fish (heart health, etc.) and the minimal to nonexistent risk of harm. For something as serious as breast cancer prevention, if an intervention carries very little risk of harm, any evidence supporting its use is sufficient.

What Kind of Fish . . . and What about Mercury?

What specific kinds of fish should you be eating, and what do I mean by "oily cold-water fish"? The reason we prefer fish from cold waters for their high omega-3 content is due to an adaptation of those species to their environment. Fish are cold-blooded, and their body temperature will approximate the temperature of the water in which they swim. Imagine the difficulty a fish near the Arctic Circle would have if its predominant body fat were butter for example. Solid at room temperature, that butter fish would not be able to move a muscle (not a great evolutionary advantage). Omega-3 fats are still liquid at very low temperatures, allowing that very cold fish to stay nice and flexible for swimming. (And it is a good reminder for you to minimize consuming fats that are solid at room temperature.)

Some examples of cold-water oily fish with high omega-3 content are:
- wild Alaskan salmon,
- sardines,
- Atlantic mackerel (not king mackerel),
- sablefish from Alaska or Canada,
- anchovies,
- farmed oysters, and
- farmed rainbow trout (one of the few times I will recommend any farmed seafood; current aquaculture practice gives this farmed fish very little contaminants and a good fat profile).

These listed are all types of seafood you can enjoy while knowing they are from sustainable fisheries with little negative impact on the environment.

Since I am recommending fish to women, I need to address pollution. The damage that is being done to our ocean's ecosystems by non-sustainable fishing practices and pollution could spell disaster for future generations of human life on our planet, and at the very least, you would like your children and grandchildren to be able to enjoy eating fish as well. [2]

Mercury in fish and its risks to pregnant women and young children is a serious concern. Women of child-bearing age should shop for and eat only those fish which are known to be low in mercury (see the Environmental Defense Fund's website for a listing). Avoid large predator fish such as shark, king mackerel and swordfish. These large fish are concentrated with toxins that have been passed all the way up the food chain.

With that said, do not use the mercury concern as a reason to avoid fish during pregnancy. The health benefits to a growing fetus that accrue when a pregnant woman eats fish are numerous. Decreased allergic disease is one, and even more profoundly important is higher levels of cognitive and social development for those children as they approach school age. Fish truly is "brain food" from the earliest stages of human development. Just eat the right type of fish.

Why wild Alaskan salmon rather than other kinds? Most Atlantic salmon found in stores and restaurants is farm raised, and there have been significant concerns brought up about pollution and contamination of farm-raised salmon with PCBs (cancer-causing chemicals). Farmed salmon is also typically lower in omega-3 fats than wild salmon.

You can get an idea of the difference between health benefits from wild versus Atlantic farm-raised salmon by looking at their meat color side-by-side in the grocery display. The farm-raised fish does not have that healthy bright-pink/orange color. I was having a discussion about fish with the butcher at my local grocery. We both commented on the color difference between wild Alaskan and farm-raised Atlantic salmon. He pointed out that even the slightly healthy color of the farmed fish was *because of colorings that were added to the fish before they arrived at the store*! You can buy frozen or canned wild Alaskan salmon year-round, but be aware that fresh wild Alaskan salmon is only available during the summer fishing season. Any fresh salmon labeled "wild Alaskan" in the winter months is a fraud, probably farmed salmon being sold at a higher price.

What if you get tired of salmon, or you are in a hurry? Sardines are the fast food of the omega-3 fish world. . . . Open the can and you are ready to enjoy.

But first, some details on why this is such a good option. One can of sardines (usually four ounces or about 120 grams) has close to 2,000 milligrams (two grams) of omega-3 fatty acids, and ounce for ounce is close to salmon in omega-3 content. Another reason to love sardines is that they are wild-caught; not in any danger of depletion from the oceans (they are rapid breeders); and they are extremely low in contaminants. Sardines can be eaten without fear of mercury or other chemicals. The Environmental Defense Fund ranks Pacific (U.S.) sardines as one of its top eco-friendly fish.

To get to know and love this marine treat, you will probably want to experiment with different brands and types. Bones versus no-bones, packed in olive oil, tomato sauce or water, you will decide your preference. Your own creativity and taste will be your best guide to enjoyment.

Choosing Your Omega 3s

What are the specific types of omega-3 fish oils we want the most? The two kinds of omega-3 fats we are most interested in are DHA (docosohexaneoic acid) and EPA (eicosopentaneoic acid). Both DHA and EPA are *essential fatty acids*, meaning that humans cannot internally manufacture these—we have to ingest them.

You get plenty of both from eating those fish we talked about, but what if you are a vegetarian? There are plenty of good vegetable sources of omega-3 fats (such as flax; see Chapter 7), but for the most part this comes as alpha-linolenic acid (ALA), not as EPA or DHA. And since humans are not a very efficient factory for transforming ALA into EPA and DHA, I typically recommend fish oil based on the science, rather than staying all vegetarian for any reason. Consider taking a fish oil capsule even if you won't eat fish. Take two grams per day as a good preventive dose, looking for brands of fish oil with the highest concentrations of EPA and DHA. If you would not consider a fish oil capsule at all, there are commercially available omega-3 supplements with high concentrations of DHA made from algae. For the purest vegetarians, these can be a good option.

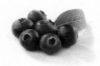

CHAPTER 7

Flax: The Big Point About a Tiny Seed

As I look through the chapters in this book that detail the specific foods I believe to be among your best allies in preventing breast cancer, flax stands out to me as perhaps the most important single food to emphasize in this particular volume. I have two reasons for saying that: one is that the data on the role of flax seed are so strong, and the other because I want this to be a food you remember.

If you are going to remember your flax seeds every day, there will have to be some reminders and lots of motivation. Why? Frankly, it is because it is not such an interesting food from a culinary or taste point of view. Flax seed, honestly, is a little boring compared to, say, wild Alaskan salmon or shiitake mushrooms.

> **If I recommend that you eat a small serving of a very plain food every day, I need to build a pretty airtight case in its favor.**

It's interesting first to consider the history of this plant and its seeds, and how for so many centuries it has been an important crop. Flax was cultivated in the ancient Middle East, including Egypt and Palestine, and its major use was turning the fibrous stalk into cloth, which we now call linen. The seed (also called linseed) was known as a useful food from very early history. The widespread use of flax fibers for cloth in Europe led to the use of the term "flaxen-haired" for young women with blond hair. (The notable cultural reference to this is Claude Debussy's musical composition "The Girl with the Flaxen Hair.")

Moving into modern times, the oil from the pressed seed (linseed oil) was turned into many products useful in the industrial chemical age. But of most interest to us today, modern herbal research has linked this tiny seed to the prevention and treatment of the root of most chronic diseases, i.e. inflammation.

At the Pendergrast household, there are two electric coffee grinders on the kitchen countertop. One is dedicated entirely to grinding flaxseed. We buy organically grown flaxseed, in bulk or pre-bagged, in the natural foods section of the grocery store. Then we keep it refrigerated or even freeze it if it won't be used for a long while.

Whenever it's time for flax seed (and that is every day, as you will see in a few moments), we take out about 2 tablespoons and grind it to powder in its dedicated grinder. It then can be sprinkled on salads, yogurt, or used in smoothies. My wife Gail prefers to eat the plain ground flax seed straight out of a spoon. Unusual, but she gets straight to the point.

Now let's look at all the reasons you will want to make flax a part of your household habits.

Flax, Algae, Fish and Humans

The more I read research articles from nutrition and medical journals, the more I am convinced that flax seeds can be a healthy part of all of our diets, men and women alike. They are an excellent source of omega-3 fatty acids, specifically alpha-linolenic acid (ALA). ALA is the natural vegetarian source of omega-3s that fish utilize to make DHA and EPA, which we ingest during that great fish dinner you started thinking about a chapter ago.

Fish, of course, do not eat flax seed, but they do enjoy algae from the ocean (which is then passed up the food chain and concentrated in larger fish), and it is the algae that is the manufacturer of the long-chain polyunsaturated fatty acids, including ALA. Fish convert ALA efficiently to EPA and DHA, which are the most important essential fatty acids for human health.

Humans do not convert ALA to EPA and DHA efficiently, which is why I recommend fish and fish oil for most people instead of solely relying on vegetarian sources of omega-3s. At the same time, it is quite true that most of us do not eat fish daily (or even close), so some vegetable sources make sense.

> **For all practical purposes, flax seed is your best vegetarian source of omega-3 fatty acids.**

Also remember: omega- 3s are healthy for your heart. They promote health in almost every body system, because they are anti-inflammatory.

Comparing Flax to Other Seeds—No Contest

Discussions routinely circulate in popular literature and websites about other seeds and their health benefits. It is true that there are many health benefits of seeds in general, and in particular pumpkin and hemp seeds deserve a close look. But they deserve a close look *not* because of their omega-3 fatty acid content, which is minimal.

When comparing the omega-3 content of popular seed or nut foods, flax far outshines its nearest competitors. One tablespoon of flax seed contains more than 3.5 grams of omega-3 fats (and recall I am recommending two tablespoons per day). By comparison, the same weight of walnuts provides 1.5 grams (roughly) of omega-3 fats, still a very nice and healthy serving, but a distant second to flax. And what about those pumpkin seed kernels? There are only about 30 milligrams of omega-3 fats in that tablespoon, and that seed will also provide a very large dose of omega-6 fats, adding further to the inflammatory ratio of high omega-6 compared to low omega-3 in the diet.

Flax Fiber for Colon and Heart Health—and Always Grind the Seeds

Flax seeds are also a good source of fiber for intestinal health, reducing constipation and the risk of diverticular disease. Some researchers believe that it is the fiber in flax seed that is most responsible for its cholesterol-lowering effect. It lowers total and LDL cholesterol but it does not lower HDL, the good cholesterol. And this fiber effect works even when the seed is ground and cooked. In fact, if the seed is not ground, you may as well not eat it.

Flax seed is covered with a very hard husk that resists digestion; this served the plant well over centuries of the nibbling of grazing animals that unknowingly replanted the seeds some days later in another location, surrounded of course by a generous heap of natural fertilizer.

Take a lesson from the goats, and don't eat your flax seed whole. Get a small electric coffee grinder and dedicate it to flax alone in your kitchen. Grind only two tablespoons at a time, and eat it fresh to avoid oxidation of the easily spoiled ALA. If your flax seed has gone rancid, you will know by the smell. Do not eat flax seed that smells like paint thinner.

Lignans Decrease Breast Cancer Risk

Perhaps the best news in the context of our search for a breast cancer prevention diet is that these little seeds have significant data supporting their role in reducing that risk. They are very high in lignans, cancer-protective compounds with a phytoestrogenic effect. This means that they have a weak ability to bind to estrogen receptors and may block some of the long-term tumor-promoting risks of natural estrogen. Laboratory and human data have shown some protective benefit against breast cancer development. (However, note that though the oil has some health benefits, flax oil itself does not contain lignans, and would not have the same cancer-protective qualities.)

In summary, the two characteristics of flax seed which are most important for breast cancer prevention are their anti-inflammatory quality (because of omega 3 oils) and the presence of protective lignans. The recommended daily dose for women is one to two tablespoons of ground flax seed per day. Keep the seeds in the refrigerator to avoid oxidation and rancidity, and only grind as much as you are going to use for one day. You can sprinkle the powder on other foods, make a smoothie or eat the powder alone (somewhat difficult when dry!).

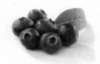

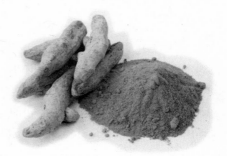

CHAPTER 8
Healthy Spices

Just as I have gained a reputation for hiding tofu and other soy foods when cooking for my unsuspecting family, I am also known for some "unusual" combinations of spices in my kitchen. Some would even say excessive spices. In my own defense, there are two simple reasons for this. One is that I enjoy spicy foods; their interesting and exotic tastes make meals resemble an international adventure. The second is that I have learned some of the medicinal properties of spices.

> **I find the thought of preventing or treating disease with the delicious foods I eat to be enticing.**

In culinary traditions around the world, spices have just those two functions. Herb gardens have been used by chefs for centuries not only for flavor but also for health and healing. And despite the fact that my family claims I have really strange preferences for recipes, I hope you will join me in discovering the wonders of spices that are both interesting and healing.

> **With this chapter, we are shifting focus slightly to introduce the concept of using spices as preventive medicine.**

Not only will you enjoy the flavor of many of the spices recommended, it is quite a remarkable added bonus that there is science to support their effectiveness in cancer prevention. Interestingly, many herbal products and spices around the world have a long oral history passed down from generation to generation, but a history that is often discredited by modern conventional medicine. Oral history is a legitimate form of scientific observation. When for generation after generation, the tribal healers have consistently noted health benefits of a spice or plant material, that painstaking and time-tested observation cannot be easily dismissed.

While I personally believe that there are many more spices with potent cancer-preventive properties than the few I will present here, this chapter will focus on ones that modern science supports in a role in breast cancer prevention.

Turmeric—Not Just for Curry Anymore

First, and perhaps most important is a spice that has well-researched anticancer properties. Turmeric imparts that characteristic yellow-orange color to Indian foods, and has a distinctive flavor. It is not highly pungent or "hot" like chili peppers, just very flavorful. The spice is the ground powder from the rhizome (underground stem) of the turmeric plant, which is closely related to ginger. It has been cultivated and used in cooking for at least 4,000 years of recorded history in India—ample time to accumulate a significant number of observations about its value to human health.

The major ingredient of turmeric powder is curcumin, an ingredient that has been the subject of medical research on breast cancer. Studies have shown that curcumin significantly slows the growth of breast cancer cells started by exposure to pesticides. And a 1997 research study[1] showed that when turmeric is used against laboratory cancer cells in combination with a soy protein called genistein, the effect was even stronger. However, at least one study has shown that the addition of curcumin to the diet *during* chemotherapy made the chemotherapy less effective because curcumin is such a strong antioxidant.

Let me be very clear in my recommendations. Based on good science, I recommend that women who are concerned with breast cancer prevention eat turmeric spice on a regular basis. Women who already have breast cancer can add it to their diet, but not during chemotherapy. Once chemotherapy is completed, adding turmeric makes good sense as a way to enhance standard treatment. If you don't enjoy the taste of turmeric, you can find it as a ground powder in capsules. While there are no standardized preventive dosing guidelines, I recommend somewhere around 500 milligrams twice daily.

Many believe that one of the reasons turmeric is a good cancer preventive is because it is such a potent anti-inflammatory (recall the discussion of inflammation, cancer and COX-2 receptors in Chapter 6, Go Fish). Turmeric inhibits an immune compound in the body called NF-kappa B; it can flare out of control in inflammatory disease states. A number of other herbs, including ginger, that are potent anti-inflammatory compounds also inhibit NF-kappa B.

Ginger—a Multi-Purpose Anti-Inflammatory

Ginger is a plant that is very closely related to turmeric, and it is another spice whose medicinal properties have been known for centuries. Ginger has the botanical name *Zingiber officinale*, indicating its "official" place in the historical pharmacy of natural medicines. The root of the plant is the part we consume, and it was first widely cultivated and used as a medicinal food in China and India. It was brought to Europe centuries ago on the early spice trade routes, and because of its value it was cultivated as a commodity on colonial islands in the Caribbean.

We know it has been used for approximately 2,000 years in traditional Chinese medicine for nausea and improving digestion. In Ayurvedic medicine, ginger has been thought to prevent heart disease and to treat arthritic complaints. It is generally seen as a "warming" remedy for illnesses and conditions associated with being cold.

In the modern era, we have learned that ginger has potent anti-inflammatory properties, reducing production of prostaglandins and leukotrienes, which circulate in higher levels in the blood during inflammatory states. Ginger is such a powerful anti-inflammatory that it may have a role in preventing the progression of Alzheimer's disease by inhibiting the activity of an inflammatory marker in the brain called TNF-alpha. [2]

Since we know that inflammation is at the root of much cancer initiation, this seems to be a promising avenue for prevention of a variety of tumors, though this approach has not been researched widely. The early research that has been done on ginger and cancer prevention has been promising. Specifically, colon and ovarian cancer have been inhibited in laboratory studies by the use of ginger and its extracts. While I have no data showing that ginger prevents breast cancer, I recommend its intake regularly with the belief that its addition to your anti-inflammatory armor could be protective, and ginger is as safe as an herb can get.

> While I personally prefer to take my medicine as food, I am frequently asked, "How much ginger should I take?" There are no definitive dosing guidelines, but if you want to take a powdered ginger extract in capsules, a minimum dose would be 250 milligrams four times daily (with meals and bedtime). If you like the crystallized ginger, one cube is probably 1,000 milligrams of ginger, and one or two a day would be a good dose. Ginger is a very safe herb with virtually no toxicity or interaction with drugs.

Rosemary—Especially with Meats

Rosemary is another spice with anti-inflammatory properties, and animal research has shown that rosemary can help inhibit the development of mammary tumors induced by chemical carcinogens. Rosemary is often used as a spice with meats, and given my general cautions about the health risks of meats (especially cooked very hot), I would recommend using rosemary frequently in marinades and seasoning mixes.

Onions and Garlic—Food or Spice?

The general class of *allium* vegetables are sometimes thought of as spices and sometimes as foods, but whether we are discussing garlic (*allium sativum*) or onions (*allium cepa*), there is no doubt that these pungent foods add spice to our kitchens. We also have well-documented data showing that garlic and onions have anticancer properties. Garlic specifically is known to reduce the risk of cancers of the esophagus, stomach and colon.

Onions are very high in a compound called quercitin. In a 1999 study, quercitin was shown to decrease the activity of the estrogen receptor in the type of breast cancer where those receptors are active. And in the *International Journal of Oncology*, a 2001 study showed that quercitin caused breast cancer cell death in a laboratory model.[3]

While population studies have been mixed (only a few studies have suggested that higher intake of *allium* vegetables lowers breast cancer risk, and many have shown no association), the scant data suggesting breast cancer risk reduction, coupled with massive amount of data for the other health benefits of garlic and onion, give me reason to unequivocally commend these spicy foods to you.

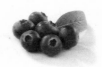

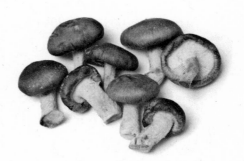

Chapter 9
Mushrooms

At any American dinner table, the appearance of mushrooms as a side dish or in a mix of vegetables is likely to divide the group in two: people who like mushrooms, and people who intensely dislike them. If you are in the latter group, I'm asking you to stay open-minded for a few moments, and you will likely find some reasons to learn to love this often misunderstood food.

Hundreds of scientific articles in the past 20 years have solidified the role of mushrooms in preventing and treating some very serious health conditions. Perhaps the greatest interest currently is their role in cancer treatment and prevention. Many different species of mushrooms have active medicinal properties, and they act on many different types of cancer. There are studies showing that mushrooms in the diet and mushroom extracts taken as medicines have activity against cancers at many body sites. But it is our specific interest today to review their role in breast cancer prevention.

What's the Good Science about Mushrooms?

Here is an abbreviated sampling of the findings of recent scientific papers on mushrooms and cancer prevention:

- An article in *The Journal of Nutrition* in 2001 discussed the effect of the lowly *white button* mushroom on lowering aromatase activity in breast tissue, thus decreasing high estrogen levels, which can promote tumor growth.[1]

- Articles in 2003 and 2004 discussed the ability of *Ganoderma* (the reishi mushroom) to prevent cancers generally, and specifically to inhibit the growth of invasive breast cancer cells. [2,3]

- There is a huge amount of science supporting the anti-cancer effect of a compound called lentinan from the *shiitake* mushroom, with citations stretching back into the 1960s; a compound called beta-D-Glucan has been isolated from the *maitake* mushroom and accounts for much of its anti-cancer effect. These work in many positive ways; of particular importance is its ability to strengthen the body's own natural immune response.

First, a Brief Caution about a Few Mushroom Types

A brief word of caution is in order. Despite the data showing that the common *button* mushrooms lower aromatase activity, which in theory could reduce breast cancer risk, you need to limit their consumption. The reason is that these mushrooms, belonging to the mushroom family *Agaricus*, contain a toxin that may be a cancer promoter and is not destroyed by most cooking.

Crimini and *portobello* mushrooms are members of the same family and share the same toxin. Most mushrooms contain some toxins, but these are usually destroyed by cooking, and become a non-issue. This may not be the case for Agaricus mushrooms, so I would minimize their consumption and enjoy other varieties.[4]

> **Another important caution: I remind you that unless you have special education and training in this area, do not harvest and eat wild mushrooms from your yard or the woods. There are mushrooms that are extremely toxic, even rapidly fatal. Leave the harvesting of mushrooms to the experts.**

And, while discussing the health benefits of cooking them, I recommend that you *never eat any mushrooms raw*. There are two reasons:

- First, recall that caution above regarding traces of toxins that are destroyed by cooking.

- Second, the nutritional benefits of mushrooms and the compounds responsible for their medical effects are tied up in the fibrous, woody structure, and would be indigestible when eaten raw. *Cooking releases these compounds so that your body can assimilate them.*

Eating Mushrooms or Swallowing Supplements?

Just as mushrooms divide people into two groups, mushrooms themselves can be divided into two groups: those which are edible and those which are not. Two of the species mentioned—*shiitake* and *maitake*—are edible and reasonably easy to find in supermarkets.

Other mushrooms with medical value are not especially edible, and will commonly be found as supplements: either as pills or alcohol-based tinctures. This includes the *reishi* mushroom, naturally so tough and woody that it is usually taken as a supplement and not eaten as food. *Cordyceps*, which has great medical value, is another mushroom that you will only find as a supplement.

Preparation Tips

In case you are not accustomed to buying and cooking mushrooms, here are a few pointers to make it simple when just beginning.

I find that reasonably fresh *shiitake* mushrooms are often available in the produce section of my local markets. Look for mushrooms with a relatively light color and not a lot of black spots, which indicate they are not as fresh. Keep them refrigerated until ready to cook, and don't wait too long and let them go bad. Break off the hard, woody stems, and only rinse them when ready to cook. Slice them into bite-size segments and use in stir-fries, soups or as a side dish of mushrooms sautéed in olive oil.

Maitake mushrooms are also excellent to eat in the same way, but you are most likely to find them dried, in a package, instead of fresh. Dried mushrooms will keep a long time in your pantry, and can be rehydrated by soaking overnight in cold water. They can then be prepared the same way you would the fresh mushrooms. Many of the other exotic mushrooms are easy to chop into soups and stir-fries. And when you think of all the good they are doing for your health, you may be surprised at how good they taste!

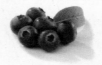

CHAPTER 10

Berries

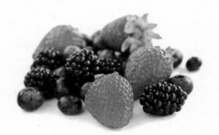

If you haven't "got it" already, you will. This chapter is where I prove to you that a cancer-prevention diet can be, and should be, loaded every day with sweet and delicious treats. I'm talking about berries here, and as much of a mix as possible. The dark reds, purples and blues are all visual evidence of something much deeper than that which meets the eye. Those vivid colors only become evident when the fruit is ripe, with the color vibrant and the fruit at the height of its sweetness. How amazing it is that we have such a signature of the perfectly ordered generosity of nature . . . a gift from the architect of the universe.

> **The pigments that show up as the colors of the berries you love are powerful anti-cancer compounds; compounds about which we are learning more as research advances.**

All of the edible berries cited below can be found in your market. They share these cancer preventing qualities. Please enjoy all of them regularly, but don't stop here—choose even more. Nature has created a smorgasbord to select from!

Strawberries

It's hard to find someone who does not love strawberries. They are a short-lived delicacy of springtime, best when fresh off the vine. In the years when my children were young, I can recall many late spring expeditions to "pick your own" strawberry farms. While filling up my little white bucket, there was an occasional berry that never made it to the bucket. Added bonuses were the occasions for my young children to learn that food comes from the earth, not from the grocery shelf!

Surrounded by a myriad of strawberry plants, I became forever grateful for the hands that pick the strawberries I find in the store. Strawberries are not scooped up by machines; they are always picked one berry at a time. And what a fabulous bonus it is that this delicious berry is also full of cancer-fighting phytochemicals!

A 2006 laboratory study demonstrated that a strawberry extract was able to decrease the rate of proliferation of breast cancer cells. And of particular interest, those researchers took the time to compare conventional versus organically grown strawberries and found that the extract from organically grown strawberries was not only higher in antioxidants, but also did a better job inhibiting the growth of the cancer cells.[1] This is consistent with a large study that looked at Chinese women and their risk of breast cancer, finding that fruit intake in general decreased risk.[2]

Like raspberries, strawberries are high in ellagic acid, an important phytonutrient that deserves some space to itself. Ellagic acid, found abundantly in many different berries, confers three cancer-fighting abilities on strawberries:

- detoxification of chemicals in the body that could cause cancer;
- antioxidant ability to prevent cellular damage by oxygen free-radicals;
- and the ability to actually slow the growth of cancer cells.

Based on this alone, wouldn't you like to have a few strawberries right now?

Raspberries

Let's move now to an even more ephemeral summer treat, the raspberry. It always amazes me that this very delicate fruit can even travel intact from the cane on which it grows and then to the market. Thankfully, it does! Raspberries are full of cancer-fighting properties.

Evidence has been mounting in research laboratories for the past 20 years about the multitude of ways that fresh fruits decrease risk of cancers of all types. And like strawberries, raspberries are an especially good source of ellagic acid. It's one of the reasons they make the list of top cancer-preventing foods.

The raspberry has been used in European herbal medicine for centuries, since at least the 1600s. It is only in recent years that advances in laboratory phytochemistry have given us the details on its potent anticancer effects. Since the fresh berries have a short harvest season, you can buy bags of frozen berries (avoid berries packed in sugar syrup) and use those as toppings or for baking. To avoid the dangers of pesticide residues, I do recommend buying organic whenever possible.

Cranberries

This is a berry you are not likely to put directly into your mouth while picking; it's much too tart for that! But the disease preventing qualities of cranberries are also impressive. They are packed with phytochemicals such as flavonols, catechins (similar to green tea), and anthocyanidin. These are powerful antioxidants which prevent oxidative damage to cells and your DNA. Adding another red berry to your menu of choices is a health strategy for reducing the likelihood of any number of chronic diseases as we age, including cancer.

As an aside, I should say a few words about the use of cranberries for the prevention of urinary infections. You need to know that cranberry juice is not effective at treating bladder infections, but it can be quite effective at preventing them. Once the infection has taken hold, it is too late for cranberries. But if you are prone to bladder infections, taking some cranberry juice (at least 4 ounces of juice, not diluted juice cocktail) every 12 hours can block the most common bacteria from adhering to the bladder wall.

Blueberries

In the east central Georgia/western South Carolina area where I live, blueberries become ready for picking in the late spring or early summer. The bushes do not mind very poor soil, so the sandy clay of this area near the Savannah River is well suited. We have four bushes just a few steps from the front door of our house—bushes I have to watch carefully, as the birds love the berries as much as we do. Dark ripe blueberries fresh off the bush are a special treat that we look forward to every spring.

We have good reasons to love them in addition to their taste. They are one of nature's most powerful sources of natural antioxidants. Dark blue fruits (blueberries and blackberries for example) are rich sources of a class of antioxidants called anthocyanins. Among the many explanations for the association between a diet higher in fresh vegetables and fruits and a lower risk of breast cancer is the well-supported theory that it is the antioxidant effect of these foods that at least in part accounts for their cancer-preventive effect.

Of all the dark fruits available for consumption, only elderberries and chokeberries (a little hard to find) exceed blueberries in anthocyanin content. This is one of the significant reasons that blueberries (no matter how you eat them) consistently rank among the highest for antioxidant capacity of all fruits measured.

A Brief Primer on Antioxidants

Let's take a moment now to consider the role of antioxidants. What do they do and why are they important? Everyone needs antioxidants because of the presence of free radicals in the body. Normal body metabolism creates free radicals every second of the day. These free radicals are the result of the normal processes of cellular metabolism, just like combustion products and "pollution" are the normal byproducts of a car engine.

Free radicals can also be the result of the body's exposure to environmental toxins (see Chapter 3, Minimizing Environmental Toxins). Whether we make them ourselves or are "attacked" from the environment, these unstable free radicals tend to damage cells and DNA, causing mutations to cells and sometimes even cancer.

> **Without a daily supply of antioxidants, the free radicals would do their damaging work unchecked.**

It is not sufficient to skip several days of eating well, then attempt to "make up for it" by eating four days worth of produce in one day, or juicing once a week instead of consuming a colorful antioxidant diet daily. Integrating berries and vegetables on a daily basis will create a great barrier to free radicals. Enjoy them freely; be consistent, making them as common as a glass of water on a hot day or as enjoyable as your favorite first beverage in the morning.

The general principle here is that a diet high in a wide variety of vegetables and fruits is a very effective strategy for cancer prevention. Since all of these berries are "high achievers" in antioxidant capacity, it makes good sense to include them in your family's diet on a regular basis—even more so when you can get them fresh and local. When berries come in season in your part of the country, take the time to find a local farmer and bring home enough to enjoy fresh and then freeze for the rest of the year. Your body will thank you.

Choosing Organic Berries is Important

And finally, choose organically grown fruits whenever possible. It is important, especially for breast cancer prevention. One of the reasons is discussed in Chapter 3, Minimizing Environmental Toxins. Specifically, pesticides are able to act as xenobiotics in the body, mimicking the hormonal action of estrogen and stimulating the growth of tumors. That is why I recommend you do all you can to avoid consuming pesticide residues as a reasonable precautionary principle.

But there's more. Remember the 2006 study cited earlier in this chapter? It showed that organically grown strawberries did a better job of inhibiting laboratory breast cancer cell lines than conventionally grown (really a nasty blow to those who still assert that organic agriculture confers no health benefits). This is actually what one would expect when you think about the growth of the fruit and the plant. Here's why:

> Organically grown vegetables and fruits are more vulnerable to attack from bugs, caterpillars and disease than conventionally grown plants; the latter are sprayed and fertilized to artificially protect them and stimulate rapid growth. *Organic plants therefore produce more of their own natural defense mechanisms in the face of that environmental stress.* Mother Nature delivers a double bonus: Those natural defense mechanisms, protective antioxidants, not only protect the plant and fruit from damage, but also protect us from environmental stress when consumed.

There are numerous studies that now support the single study cited above. We know now more broadly that antioxidant content of organic produce is generally higher across the board than conventional produce. The question arises: should you buy only organic produce? After all, it is usually quite a bit more expensive. Here is what I would do: keep up to date on the most contaminated produce items,[3] and insist on organic only for the top 10 contaminated foods. Because this list may change over time, I have included a current website where you can keep up with the latest information, the Shopper's Guide to Pesticides, *www.FoodNews.org.*

For example, since conventional strawberries are near the top of the list in pesticide-laden foods, this is a food you should always buy organic; you can enjoy those strawberries, knowing your health is worth every bite. But conventional blueberries, one of the powerhouses of the berry group, ranks as number 32 on the current list. You are safe choosing conventional blueberries if the cost of organic is prohibitive. Or better yet, grow your own!

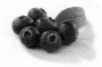

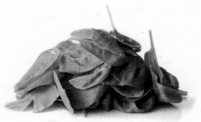

CHAPTER 11
Dark Green Leafy Vegetables

A general strategy for reducing cancer risk and specifically breast cancer risk is to maximize the variety of vegetables and fruits consumed daily. Here, another group of vegetables is special enough to deserve its own chapter: green, leafy vegetables. (Recall that the cruciferous vegetables had their own spotlight in Chapter 5, Cruciferous Vegetables). Green leafy vegetables deserve your appreciation not only for their disease-fighting capacity, but also for their delicious way of bringing joy to your senses in a meal!

Antioxidants from Green Leafy Vegetables

The reasons that vegetables make cancer less likely are still being discovered—they are even more in number than the variations in color you can get on your plate. One important role they play is to provide a steady stream of antioxidants into the body. You need antioxidants because of the presence of free radicals in the body, and recall that normal body metabolism creates free radicals every second (see the previous chapter on berries).

The two antioxidants I want to emphasize in the context of green leafy vegetables are folate (folic acid) and carotenoids (natural precursors of vitamin A, including beta-carotene and lutein):

Studies on dietary reduction of breast cancer risk give special importance to the roles of carotenoids and folic acid. A study

89

published in the *Journal of the National Cancer Institute* in 1999 showed that the more alpha-carotene, beta-carotene, and lutein/zeaxanthin women consumed from foods, the lower their breast cancer risk.[1] These are natural carotenoids found in high levels in carrots, dandelion greens, red peppers, collards, chard and other green leafy vegetables.

Chard—Colorful Disease Prevention that Tastes Great

Because variety is so important to your diet, let me encourage you to get to know chard, which is not one of the most popular vegetables. Chard is especially high in natural carotenoids and is also high in vitamins C, K, and the mineral, magnesium. Although not high in folate like other green leafy vegetables, it is an exceptionally good source of the natural carotenoids, which promote so many aspects of health by their powerful antioxidant capacity. One cup of cooked chard provides more than double the daily requirement for vitamin A, without any risk of overdose. This is because it is the natural form, not as preformed vitamin A that is found in less expensive vitamin pills.

Chard may be found in groceries as several different varieties: red, yellow, or rainbow-colored, referring to the color of the thick stem. The leaves are large, green and slightly curly. The nutritional benefits are the same for all; so the color you choose is really a matter of how you would like your dinner to appear.

Don't get hung up about which type to choose, as the general principle still applies: the higher your diet is in all fruits and vegetables, the lower your cancer risk is across the board.

Spinach—So Much Better than You Remember

While chard is very high in natural carotenoids but not very high in folate, there is a more familiar dark green leaf that is a folate superstar. Spinach is near the top of the list of foods that are high in folate. Research published in the *Journal of the National Cancer Institute* in 2003 demonstrated that a higher level of folate in the blood is associated with a lower risk of breast cancer, especially among women who drink alcohol.[2] Folate is an important factor in the synthesis of DNA, and if folate is deficient, DNA is more likely to be made with an incorrect code in the nucleic acid sequence, making cancer more likely. An added bonus for spinach is that it provides high amounts of natural carotenoids in every serving.

Spinach can be enjoyed in countless ways. I prefer to buy fresh organic spinach leaves, and wash them thoroughly before cooking because they tend to pick up bits of good organic soil before leaving the farm! By weight, cooked or frozen spinach has about 75 percent as much folate as the fresh vegetable, but because it cooks down so much, a cup of cooked spinach has much more folate than a cup of raw spinach. If you enjoy a good spinach salad, make it a nice big one; if you prefer it cooked, you can be assured that every bite is full of cancer-preventing folate.

Asparagus—Let's Hear It for an Overlooked Friend

I'm going to sneak a vegetable "underdog" into this chapter for two reasons. Yes, I know it's not a "green leafy." But promoting asparagus will definitely appeal to those of you who are always pulling for the underdog, as asparagus in the U.S. ranks near dead-last in per capita consumption of a long list of common fresh produce items in USDA data.

My first reason for including asparagus here is because of how much I want you to expand your list of produce items you eat regularly, and this really wonderful food just gets neglected too often. Recall that one of the foundational principles for disease prevention through foods is to consume a wide variety of fresh vegetables and fruits. It is important to look very literally for a rainbow of colors in your plant foods.

This strategy of variety assures a wide mix of phytonutrients, which work together in a synergistic way to neutralize toxins in the body, optimize immune function and promote health at the level of the cell. To get straight to the point, adding an unpopular vegetable to your plate breaks you out of a boring rut of always eating the same foods . . . and it expands your horizon of choices.

Second, let's look at the nutritional profile of asparagus. Per serving, asparagus is one of the highest vegetable sources of folate (folic acid). When both are cooked, it is even higher than spinach . . . surprise! A critical role of folate is the prevention of incorrect DNA sequences. Another is that folate also plays a very important role in bringing down blood levels of homocysteine. Homocysteine is an independent risk factor for heart disease and stroke. Not only is asparagus an important part of the vegetable team in reducing your risk of breast cancer, add cardiovascular disease prevention to the list of credits for this neglected veggie.

Asparagus is also an excellent source of vitamin A precursors (carotenoids); when carotenoid levels in the blood increase, risk of cancer goes down. Like many dark green vegetables, asparagus is loaded with Vitamin K, important for healthy bones. Ranking very high in vegetable sources of omega-3 fatty acids, it rounds out its role as an important anti-inflammatory vegetable.

Kale—A Leafy Brassica Doing Double Duty

Kale is next on my list of green leafy vegetables you can love for good taste and disease prevention. It had a brief mention in Chapter 5, Cruciferous Vegetables, but it deserves its own moment of fame here with its green, leafy look-alikes. While it is a dark green leaf, it is unique among those I have emphasized. Kale is a member of the *Brassica* family of vegetables (cruciferous vegetables), and even though it does not look like its more famous cousins (broccoli, cauliflower and cabbage), it shares some of their best nutritional benefits.

Unlike broccoli, kale does not form a head, and remains a green leafy plant with somewhat curly leaves. It is a cool season garden vegetable, and many home gardeners have traditionally planted kale and other cool season greens for a fall crop. Many believe that kale tastes better when it is harvested after the first frost.

Just a quick look at the nutritional content of kale is enough to put this wonderful vegetable near the top of your list. One cup of cooked kale provides your entire day's supply of vitamin A (as natural carotenoids), more than 17,000 units; and it provides more than 50 milligrams of vitamin C. This combination of vitamins A and C makes kale an antioxidant powerhouse, a great ally in your body's process of cleaning up toxic reactive oxygen species (free radicals).

Just one cup of kale also provides a tremendous amount of vitamin K, more than 1,000 micrograms, which is very important for bone health and preventing excess bleeding. (Caution, however: If you are on prescription blood thinners like warfarin, you should avoid kale or talk with your doctor about it, as it would interfere with your medication and make clotting more likely). Kale is also a terrific vegetable source of omega-3 fatty acids; a cup has more than 130 milligrams (a good reminder that one does not always have to eat fish to get healthy fats). And it provides more than two grams of dietary fiber, good for intestinal health and also the heart.

This overall profile of antioxidants, healthy fats and fiber make this a food that is highly anti-inflammatory, good for prevention of disease and cooling down the fires of inflammatory states in the body such as chronic pain and arthritis.

It is important to note, like its *Brassica* cousins, kale is high in indole-3-carbinol (I3C), which seems to have a protective effect against the development of breast cancer. And one final bonus: One cup contains nearly 100 milligrams of calcium, adding another bone-healthy benefit to this versatile green. If you have not already learned to enjoy this delicious vegetable, it is time you did. The green, leafy vegetables are the "gold" of the nutritional spectrum.

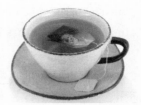

CHAPTER 12
Tea—White, Green, and Black

Tea, after water, is the most popular beverage in the world, far surpassing even coffee and sodas, and that's a good thing. All tea comes from the same plant, *Camellia sinensis*, and the varieties (white, green, oolong and black) are the result of how the leaves are processed.

> **So-called "red tea" or rooibos is not actually tea, but an infusion of a plant native to South Africa. Parenthetically, rooibos has its own health benefits, but it is not tea and will not be considered here. There are of course many other herbal teas or infusions of plants with a history of social or medicinal use, such as chamomile or ginger, but technically these also should not be called tea.**

For this chapter, I reserve that very exclusive verbal property—tea—to the hot water extract of the leaves of the shrub *Camellia sinensis*. Whether white, green, black or oolong, all tea is also healthy, but research has demonstrated some differences in benefits.

Black, Green and White—What's the Difference?

The leaves of green tea are processed less than black tea (which is oxidized and heated). The result is that green tea has exceptionally high levels of antioxidants, notably one called EGCG (epigallocatechin gallate for you chemists; it is a type of flavonoid).

White tea is processed even less than green tea. It gets its name because at the time of harvest, the new tea leaves are still curled up and covered with a fine white hair. All white tea is hand harvested at that early stage of growth, and is therefore more expensive than other teas. The leaves are allowed to dry naturally and are minimally heated to stop oxidation.

The best white teas are loose leaf rather than in bags, and the tea has a slightly sweet and pleasant flavor, and not at all "grassy" like some green teas. But if you could see and identify the flood of molecules and the complex mix of natural compounds that pours out of those leaves into your cup as they steep in the hot water, that's when you would get really excited.

Antioxidants in Tea and What They Do

Volumes of research have documented the health benefits of EGCG as found in green tea. Analysis has consistently shown that white tea also provides very high levels of EGCG. Some research literature suggests that white tea may even have higher cancer-preventing ability in laboratory experiments than green tea.

The antioxidants in tea have been thoroughly studied, and in addition to their cancer-preventing qualities, have been shown to inhibit oxidation of LDL cholesterol; oxidation of LDL is an important step on the road to development of heart disease and stroke. Laboratory studies have shown that EGCG slows the growth of breast cancer cells, even cells that have become resistant to some types of chemotherapy.

The cancer inhibitory effects of tea have been well studied, and are certainly due to a synergistic effect of the multiple compounds from the leaf—more than just EGCG or any single antioxidant. This is why I am certain that your best health strategy with regard to tea is to drink it as a whole food, and not to rely on any extracts found in pills.

Why Do We Need Antioxidants?

I cannot emphasize enough the importance of antioxidants in this discussion of tea. Just as we reviewed in Chapter 10, Berries, remember that all animals that breathe and depend on oxygen for life (that includes you and me) are constantly producing reactive oxygen species as a result of the metabolic chemical reactions in our cells. That creates a great need for antioxidants even without any exposure to environmental toxins (which create additional oxidant stress on the body).

These "free radicals" (or oxidants) are named "free" because they are inherently chemically unstable and need to chemically bond with other compounds or steal electrons from other molecules in order to be stabilized. This process of free radicals stealing electrons is damaging to our cells and DNA, and can make it more likely that there will be errors in replication of those cells, possibly leading to cancer.

Antioxidants come into the picture by acting like little molecules on a scavenger hunt. Their job is to find as many free radicals as possible and bind to them, rendering them harmless. All plants that are edible to humans have some antioxidant activity, but tea is one of the stars. Its very high antioxidant activity comes from a class of flavonoids called catechins, of which EGCG is the best studied.

Tea—Real Food for Real Cancer Prevention

This is all good news, and suggests that green tea intake may be a helpful adjunct to conventional treatment for breast cancer. What about prevention? When it comes to cancer prevention strategies, green or white tea is on par with the best dietary strategies we have discussed so far. There is very good laboratory evidence that green tea (EGCG) can inhibit the development of breast cancer by suppressing tumor-associated fatty acid synthase.

Additionally, one very interesting study (*American Journal of Clinical Nutrition,* 2007) looked at the effect of combined soy protein and tea as a cancer prevention strategy (specifically preventing breast and prostate cancer).[1] The conclusion: Green tea and soy together may work as a cancer prevention strategy because they also work to reduce the expression of the *metabolic syndrome* (abdominal obesity, elevated levels of insulin and other hormones that may promote tumor growth and heart disease). This study clarifies how obesity and breast cancer are linked; at the same time demonstrating that a specific dietary intervention (soy and tea) can help to reduce both.

While the laboratory evidence linking tea consumption to cancer risk reduction has been compelling, large-scale epidemiologic studies in living human beings have been less conclusive. I believe that this points mainly to the difficulty of doing reductionist research in large populations where the answers to life's questions never boil down to a single ingredient, single food, single drink or single lifestyle habit.

We humans are more than just the mathematical sum of all those things. There are dynamic interactions between all of our lifestyle choices that science will never be able to fully tease apart and say, "See! There's the culprit right there!" A holistic rather than a reductionist model makes more sense to me, in which we take as much of the good that is known regarding prevention, pile it into our lives all at once and not worry about "which one is making the difference." Collectively, they do the job.

Health Claims of Popular "Tea" Beverages—Be Skeptical

Another point I need to make about tea before leaving this chapter has to do with the problems of convenience marketing of food products and the exploitation of health claims. Instant iced tea has virtually no catechin antioxidants, but you can be sure that the purveyors of that beverage would like to ride the coattails of the health-related popularity of tea. If you want iced tea, brew up a pot of black or green tea, and add ice. It will still have significant antioxidant effect even though some of the antioxidant compounds adhere to the ice.

Perhaps even worse than instant tea, is the new phenomenon of ready-to-drink tea in plastic bottles.

> **The "green tea" that is now rivaling sodas and bottled water and being sold by the case in 16-ounce or 20-ounce plastic bottles, is not something I would recommend.**

The second ingredient present after water is high fructose corn syrup, which may completely negate the possible health benefits of the small amount of surviving green tea in that highly processed bottled product. That spike in blood sugar will not only promote obesity, but is also promoting inflammation!

How to prepare a really good cup of tea

Place one teaspoon of loose green tea leaves in the bottom of a glass measuring cup (Pyrex or other heat resistant), and pour eight ounces of very hot but not boiling water over them. Use filtered water that tastes good; bad water makes bad tea.
Avoid pouring boiling water on green tea, since it "cooks" the leaves and destroys some of their delicate flavor. Let it steep for two minutes and not longer if you want to prevent some of the bitterness. Most of the health-promoting antioxidants are already in the water after two minutes. You can then pour it through a strainer into your favorite teacup.

Add to the health benefits of this experience by drinking it slowly, giving yourself some space for quiet breathing or peaceful music.

For more really interesting information on tea's history, the differences between types, and other recipes, I recommend *http://www.inpursuitoftea.com*

PART 3

Foods to Avoid

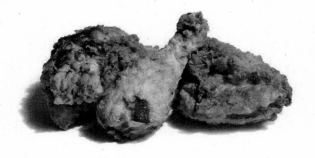

There is definitely a part of me that would like to avoid writing this section. It would be ideal if we could simply focus on the good foods that you can eat to reduce risk of breast cancer. And that was the intent of Part 2, *Foods for Breast Health*, to give you some delicious and strong allies in the prevention campaign. But you may recall in Part 1, *General Principles for Cancer Prevention*, that there was mention of toxins to avoid, and environmental risks to guard against. It is necessary at this time to spell those cautions out more clearly, and make sure that you know the dangers that are all around you in 21st century America.

Unfortunately, there are some very common cultural habits centering on food and drink that make breast cancer more likely. The ones I want most to emphasize are the ones that are not only the most common, but also the ones you can do something about. This does not mean you can never drink alcohol or enjoy charcoal-grilled meat. I hope you recall in the general principles of cancer prevention discussed in the Introduction that any dietary changes you make, move you either in the direction of higher or lower risk—there are no absolutes. I just want you to have the information, and to hear my best professional recommendations, then make your own decisions.

> **Food is still good, still to be enjoyed, and we can take sufficient precautions so that eating is not accompanied by any fear.**

This short section is divided into two parts. The first deals with traditional foods that humans have lived with for centuries, but still increase risk of breast cancer. It focuses on what we know about grilled meats and alcohol. The second part looks at foods and food additives that have only been a part of our diet for the past 50 plus years, coming on the scene with the advent of modern food science and industrial agriculture.

Foods to Avoid will not claim to cover all of the possible environmental toxins or food additives that can increase risk of breast cancer, only those that are most commonly encountered and the avoidance of which will allow you to significantly reduce risk.

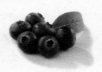

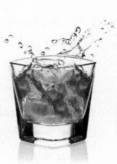

Chapter 13
Some Traditional Foods

Alcohol

As a practicing pediatrician, I have had countless discussions with kids and parents over the years about alcohol use. Most of these have been in the context of checkups during the teen years, helping kids negotiate the perilous waters of risk-taking behavior and avoiding under-age drinking. Advising parents how to discuss and model responsible alcohol use in the family has also been a frequent conversation in the office, and I confess that it is often tricky to negotiate.

In a family where very moderate and responsible alcohol use is modeled by parents, what do you tell a child who comes home from 2nd grade saying, "We had a class on drugs today at school, and they said alcohol is a drug . . . so why does Daddy drink beer?" These are very important conversations for parents and children, especially since underage drinking in teens is the root of so many injuries and deaths.

Yet even in a medical office, we don't often discuss the other potential hazards of alcohol use such as cancer risk. First, let's set it in a broader context.

The Big Picture

Alcohol has played an important role in human history since before historical records were kept. Religious ceremonies, family gatherings, cultural celebrations—such as the change of seasons or the bringing in

105

of the harvest—all were made memorable and special by the use of alcohol in drinks. While it may not have been specifically articulated in all these activities and celebrations from antiquity, it's clear that the altered state of consciousness brought about by drinking alcohol was—and is—the reason for its inclusion in special events in human affairs.

There's no doubt there is a positive side to this when alcohol is enjoyed in moderation. It also is self-evident, but needs to be said nonetheless; there is a dark side to alcohol's use in the human family. Interpersonal violence, accidental injury and neglect of what's important in relationships can all result from irresponsible use of alcohol. Abusive use of alcohol also carries its acute and long-term health risks. Among the health risks from even short-term excessive use of alcohol are:

- Dangerous inflammation of the pancreas;
- Erosion and bleeding in the stomach and esophagus; and (less commonly),
- Death from acute intoxication.

Long-term heavy use, of course, can lead to liver damage, cirrhosis and liver failure. All of these things are not news to anyone. They are emphasized here as a reminder of why I never recommend beginning to use alcohol for its health benefits because of the health risks from even short-term excessive use if one does not already drink.

Benefits of Alcohol Use

Did I say health benefits of alcohol? Yes, it has become clear in recent years that for most people, moderate alcohol use has a salutary effect, especially on heart health. This was first observed as an epidemiological fact when researchers were looking at patterns of eating that prevented heart disease. The Lyon Study[1] was famous for clarifying the importance of the so-called Mediterranean diet in prevention of heart disease. Persons living around Lyon, France, were observed to have a much lower rate of heart disease when following a traditional way of eating, which included lots of fresh produce, whole grains, limited amounts of dairy and meat, and a glass of wine with dinner.

Researchers continued to look into that association and initially attributed the benefit to antioxidants such as resveratrol in red wines. There is no doubt that resveratrol and other antioxidants from grapes play an important role, but further studies have made it clear that the heart-healthy benefits of the glass of wine with dinner are not limited to wine—red or white. It appears that any alcohol in the same moderate amount will reduce risk of heart disease.

The latest data we have suggest the following: Men who drink one or two drinks a day (A four-ounce glass of wine, a 12-ounce beer, or a 1.5-ounce serving of distilled spirits is the definition of a "drink" in this case.), and women who consume at most one drink per day reduce their risk of heart attack.[2]

> **Drinking *more* than a drink a day can raise the risk of heart disease in several serious ways.**

While the potential to reduce heart disease risk with alcohol may be tantalizing, the significant downside from alcohol use seems so dangerous that I do not include alcohol use in my health recommendations. Over all, health-wise, it doesn't make sense for persons who do not already drink or who have a family history of alcohol abuse or dependence.

Alcohol and Cancer Risk

How significant is alcohol use with regard to breast cancer risk? Alcohol has been found to be a causative factor in many different types of cancer, including colon, mouth and throat, liver and breast. In addition to its other cancer-causing mechanisms, there is a specific way that alcohol increases risk of breast cancer. You may recall from an earlier discussion that there is an enzyme in the body called aromatase. Aromatase enhances the conversion of other steroid hormones into estrogen, and higher long-term exposure to estrogen increases risk of breast cancer. Alcohol increases the activity of aromatase in the body.

> **Alcohol, in general, increases cancer risk, and specifically increases breast cancer risk because of increasing aromatase activity.**

Is there a safe threshold that I can recommend below which women can enjoy moderate alcohol use and not be concerned about increasing risk of breast cancer? Unfortunately, the answer is no. It seems that there is a "dose-response" relationship between alcohol use and breast cancer risk in women.

Dose-response means that for any given amount of alcohol consumed, the risk of breast cancer increases proportionately, and the increasing risk starts when consumption moves above zero. For reference, the very careful analysis of multiple independent studies summarized in the AICR 2007 report concluded that a woman who consumes five drinks per week increases her risk of breast cancer by five percent.[3] At higher levels of consumption, risk is much greater, so a woman who has two or more drinks per day increases her risk of breast cancer by more than 40 percent.[4]

For clarity, remember how we defined population levels of risk (principles we discussed in the Introduction). On average, out of a group of 100 US women, 13 will develop breast cancer at some time. A 40 percent increase in risk means this: Of a group of 100 women who consume at least two alcoholic drinks per day, 18 will develop breast cancer (since 18 is 40 percent more than 13). It does not mean that 40 percent of women consuming two drinks per day will get breast cancer.

To me, increasing the odds from 13 percent to 18 percent is a gamble you don't want to take. There's no real benefit from that much alcohol consumption, and I cannot think of a woman who would knowingly move herself into a group in which many more women are likely to develop cancer.

My Recommendation

What do I recommend to you regarding alcohol?

1. If you already enjoy drinking, you may continue to do so with minimal increase in your risk of breast cancer by having no more than one drink per day and preferably no more than five drinks per week (and these drinks cannot be all at the same sitting!).

2. If you do not already drink, don't start. There are plenty of other less risky ways to improve heart health.

3. Avoid alcohol use altogether if you have a personal or family history of alcohol abuse or dependence, or any history of liver disease such as hepatitis.

Grilled or Fried Meats

If you are a vegetarian, you can skip this section. That is, unless you are a vegetarian on a mission to bring meat eaters into your group. If so, this section will give you some convincing ammunition against eating meat. But not a blanket prohibition on meat, only a caution that certain ways of cooking meats add to breast cancer risk significantly.

The Chemistry Lab on Your Grill

When it comes to cancer risk, there are two chemicals of interest formed by high temperature cooking of meat. One is a group of chemicals called polycyclic aromatic hydrocarbons. The chemical structure of these molecules consists of a set of connected rings of carbon atoms with hydrogen atoms attached. If you look at a traditional drawing of their structures in a chemistry text, they are actually geometrically interesting. But don't let appearance fool you; these are dangerous compounds with a potential for inducing cancerous mutations in cells by damaging DNA.

The other chemical problem with meats cooked very hot is a group (maybe we should call it a "gang") called heterocyclic amines. These two groups of chemicals are related to each other and both are linked to increased risk of cancer.

How do polycyclic aromatic hydrocarbons get into your meat in the first place? This is primarily the result of the charring process when a meat is cooked at very high temperature. A flame-grilled steak hot off the grill may taste great, but the extremely high heat on the surface of the meat causes blackening. That blackening indicates a change in the structures of the molecules in that food, and cancer-causing chemicals are the result.

Polycyclic aromatic hydrocarbons become attached to meat by incomplete burning—charring—of the surface (such as over a wood or charcoal grill). However, the second class (or "gang") of cancer causing compounds, heterocyclic amines, are formed in meat that is simply cooked at a very high temperature, such as broiling or frying.

There are ways to still enjoy meat without the polycyclic aromatic hydrocarbons or heterocyclic amines however. Slower cooking at a lower temperature is one way. Another way is simply to avoid cooking a steak "well done."

> **When cooking beef, medium or medium-rare is a healthier choice of "done-ness."**

There was a large study of women that looked at breast cancer risk as a function of how women preferred to order their steaks cooked, and the women who most often chose "well-done" had higher risk of breast cancer. [5,6] This suggests that the significant toxic exposure from grilled meat is not something unusual or that it only occurs in unusual situations; it is a function of the common food choices with which we are all faced.

By the way, the presence of cancer-causing chemicals from charred meat is not only a property of beef steak, but can be true of any meat, poultry or fish that becomes charred during cooking at high temperature. Of course, it is very important for other health reasons to thoroughly cook poultry and pork, but it is best done slowly by baking or roasting, or letting it cook at low heat, for example, in a crock pot all day.

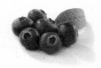

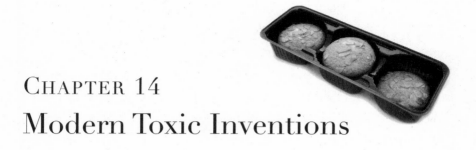

CHAPTER 14
Modern Toxic Inventions

Alcohol and grilled meats have been a part of the human diet for longer than there are historical records, and countless generations of women have enjoyed them in moderation without suffering ill effects. Though modern research has demonstrated that these confer an increased risk of breast cancer on women, their long historical precedent suggests to me a less ominous role than some of the more modern toxins we will now discuss.

Trans-fats—We Were So Wrong

The first of these unnatural foods, an invention of modern food science which turned out to be completely unsafe, is trans-fats. And the really devilish part of the story of trans-fats is how they came to be a part of our food supply in the first place.

Trans-fats first became widely available in the food supply with the gradually increasing preference for margarine over butter in the mid-1900s. For reasons that are not clear, the late 1800s saw a demand for the manufacture of "artificial butter." Parallel to the rise in the chemical manufacturing industry and the 20th century faith in science to lead humanity to a brighter future, this time in history also saw the widespread introduction of infant formulas meant to be equal or superior to human milk.

Of course, we now know that no infant formula can match human breast milk for human babies, but bottle-feeding and margarine (the name given to the "artificial butter") were just two examples of how faith in science and technologies led to the widespread adoption of certain societal trends around food.

Parenthetically, I cannot count the number of times in my practice of pediatrics that I have seen a child whose health problems were directly a result of a mother's decision to feed with cow-milk-based formula instead of her own milk. And not only would it have been better for her child, her long term breast health would have improved as well, including a lower risk of breast cancer.

> **I hope you appreciate as I do the symmetry and harmony of this scientific fact: breast feeding your baby lowers your risk of breast cancer.**

An in-depth discussion of the science of breast feeding and its benefits is beyond the scope of this book, and it is certainly not the intent of this chapter. But it is too important to pass over completely. While I am strongly emphasizing the importance of feeding yourself real foods instead of chemically modified food products, you now know that the choice to feed your infant its best real food also protects your breast health. At least one reason for this fact is that breastfeeding inhibits production of estrogen by the ovaries, decreasing a woman's overall lifetime estrogen exposure.

Margarine—A Technical Triumph and a Public Health Mistake

Margarine was the solution to the problem of how to make vegetable oil roughly the same texture and spreadable quality as butter. The manufacturers needed something that could be spread on bread and melt at about the same temperature, or to be used in cooking. The way to create such a product out of liquid vegetable oil was the process of hydrogenation. If you add enough hydrogen atoms to a polyunsaturated vegetable oil (such as corn oil) to completely fill up the chain and get rid of the double bonds, the product becomes a saturated fat, fully hydrogenated and hard at room temperature. If you add fewer hydrogen atoms, it does not become completely saturated and may be softer and more spreadable. But in the partial hydrogenation process, some of the chemical bonds between carbon atoms twist in an unnatural way, making a rigid, straight fatty acid instead of a curved and flexible fatty acid. The rigid straight fat molecule with the unnatural twist is called a trans-fat. Any margarine by the nature of its manufacturing process is full of trans-fats. This was thought for many decades to be healthier than butter because it was not completely saturated.

But this "artificial butter" still faced an uphill battle for societal acceptance. The dairy industry saw the economic threat and fought back. One way this played out was in legal bans on selling yellow margarine in most U.S. states in the middle 20th century. Margarine is naturally white, and not very appealing to look at compared to the creamy yellow of butter. In an attempt to make sure consumers did not confuse margarine with butter, laws were passed forbidding companies from putting color in the margarine at the factory.

Unfortunately for the dairy industry and the health of the public, this did not stop the thirst of 20th century Americans for "modern" foods. My father was one of scores of children in the 1930s whose kitchen chore was to mix the yellow food dye into the white margarine before home use. Eventually the laws forbidding the sale of yellow margarine were repealed, and by the 1950s, margarine was outselling butter by touting claims of better health from decreased saturated fat intake.

To put these unsubstantiated health claims, solely for the purpose of marketing, in context, recall that the 1950s still saw cigarette companies making health claims for their products as well. In fact, starting in the late 1940s, tobacco companies often used doctors in their advertisements. Knowing what we know about tobacco, it's easy to be a bit skeptical about the mid-20th-Century health claims of margarine.

> **It is wise to be skeptical of health claims on any food packages. Remember, they are placed there for only one reason: to sell more product.**

Trans-fats—Here, There and Everywhere

The next and most widespread way trans-fats have made their way into the American pantry is through the use of partially hydrogenated vegetable oils in packaged baked goods. This solved another tough problem for food manufacturers wanting to stock store shelves with prepackaged baked goods that would last long enough and not become rancid shortly after purchase.

Take the example of a commercially available cookie that uses vegetable oil in the recipe, for which the manufacturer can keep costs down and also claim to be healthier ("no saturated fats!"). That's fine for a short time, but polyunsaturated oils like vegetable oil oxidize fairly rapidly at room temperature and exposure to air. Oxidized oil has a characteristic rancid smell that people recognize as "gone bad." Once again, chemical food science came to the rescue and manufacturers began using partially hydrogenated vegetable oils instead of plain liquid oils. The resulting products have a longer shelf life, taste fresh longer, and everyone wins. From the grocer, to the trucking company, to the manufacturers, to the suppliers of raw materials, to the stockholders . . . and to . . . oh, yes . . . all but the consumers.

That's all of us. We lost on this one, and the health of America mirrors it.

Regulation of Trans-Fats—Good Idea, but Watch the Fine Print

The use of partially hydrogenated oils became ubiquitous in packaged baked goods and thus introduced trans-fats into the population at large. This continues to be an issue, even after the U.S. Food and Drug Administration began requiring food manufacturers to state the trans-fat content of their products in 2003. This was a good move by the FDA, and finally made public acknowledgment of what many public health experts had been warning about for years—that trans-fats were dangerous (especially for heart health). But the FDA left a significant loophole in the regulation. Any company (at the time of this writing) is allowed to make a "No Trans-Fat" or "Zero Grams Trans-Fat" claim on the label *if there are fewer than 500 milligrams of trans-fat per serving.* You could argue from a sort of warped mathematical perspective that this makes sense because we are just "rounding down." But from a health perspective it does not help, because consumers can be easily misled.

> **I encourage all my patients to read the "nutrition facts" panel on the back of the package instead of the advertising claims on the front. If at any point in the ingredient list the words "hydrogenated" or "partially hydrogenated oils" appear, that indicates the presence of trans-fats. Put the product back on the store shelf!**

Trans-fats can also be created in the process of deep-frying foods, and are therefore quite prevalent in restaurants that reuse their oils for frying fast foods. Ordering foods that have been deep-fried in a restaurant is not only hazardous because of the sheer amount of fat consumed, but also because by virtue of repeated use, it has been chemically altered.

Agricultural Chemicals in Food

Modern toxic inventions can show up in our food because manufacturers put them there on purpose (e.g. trans-fats) or because their presence is an accidental by-product of the chemical agricultural industry. Since World War II, agricultural production in the United States has been increasingly dependent on chemical fertilizers and pesticides. These were a natural outgrowth of the scientific technological exuberance of the mid-20th century, an era that saw great advances in our quality of life and in our capabilities because of science and engineering.

The use of science and technology to modify agricultural production was only one part of this very widespread cultural phenomenon of the years immediately after World War II in the United States. There was an unbridled optimism that technological fixes could improve upon nature. Along with that came an almost inevitable blindness to the unintended consequences of relying too heavily on chemical agriculture for food production. Activists and visionaries such as Rachel Carson (author of *Silent Spring*) and J. I. Rodale (founder of *Organic Gardening Magazine* in 1942) spoke out early on this topic, but were not widely appreciated during their lifetimes. Their foresight is much more widely appreciated now.

What are the problems with conventionally produced foods? Minimizing toxins was discussed in Chapter 3, Minimizing Environmental Toxins; the following discussion will be a brief reminder of specific foods to avoid in order for you to keep exposure to toxic chemicals to a minimum. The specific exposures considered here are those which I believe are especially pertinent to breast cancer risk, including:
- pesticide residues in produce,
- plastics from packaging leaching into foods;
- the presence of cancer-causing chemicals such as PCBs in the food chain (especially in fish);
- and hormones added to the meat and milk supply.

Pesticides and Breast Cancer Risk

At this time, I believe there is enough evidence to sound a note of caution on the possible association with pesticides on foods and breast cancer. Remember that pesticides may act as xenoestrogens when they bind to estrogen receptors in the body (specifically the breast) and cause those receptors to become active, as if there were higher levels of estrogen circulating. The longer and higher a woman's cumulative exposure to estrogen over her lifetime (even natural estrogen made by her own ovaries), the higher her breast cancer risk.

Though the data are scant, the potential for xenoestrogens from pesticides to promote breast tumors suggests the need for a precautionary approach. Do not knowingly expose yourself to a substance about which there is reasonable concern when you have an alternative.

While buying organically grown produce is more costly, one way to approach the expense issue is to be selective in choosing organic foods. Only choose to replace those produce items that are the most contaminated when grown conventionally.

> You can significantly reduce your toxic burden by purchasing organic items only for those most contaminated foods in the list published by the Environmental Working Group (*http://www.FoodNews.org*).

Currently, this includes strawberries, peaches, apples, bell peppers and many others of my favorite fruits and vegetables, which, I should add, I now choose only to buy organic.

Another Caution about Plastics and PCB's

Similar to the xenoestrogens from pesticides, compounds that can stimulate estrogen receptors can also enter the body through exposure to some plastics, such as when foods are placed in a microwave oven in a plastic container and the plastic compounds leach into the food. This caution is not really about a food to avoid but a concern about the way foods are packaged.

My precautionary principle here is to avoid cooking in plastic containers and not to store food in plastic. This includes bottled water, which is transported long distances in often hot conditions, giving ample opportunity for chemicals to leach into the water.

There are solid data showing that polychlorinated biphenyls (PCBs) pose a risk to breast health. One of the easiest ways to reduce exposure to PCBs is to know which fish are likely to be contaminated and choose instead, other, healthy fish.

Refer to the Seafood Selector from the Environmental Defense Fund at *www.EDF.org* to stay up to date on how to choose fish without PCBs. Farm-raised (Atlantic) salmon is currently one of the fish types known to be an unsafe source of PCBs, and I suggest for breast cancer risk reduction that you avoid those fish. When looking for a delicious salmon meal with high omega-3 fatty acids, consume only wild Alaskan salmon instead.

Hormones in Meat and Milk

The use of hormones in dairy and meat production also provokes my concern. The use of rBGH (recombinant bovine growth hormone) in dairy cattle leads to higher levels of insulin-like growth factor, or IGF-1. Good science has shown that IGF-1 is a tumor growth promoter. This means that any set of mutated cells that is growing out of control tends to multiply faster in the presence of IGF-1.

For something as important as breast cancer prevention, I believe this is reason enough to insist on consuming only dairy products that have not come from cows treated with rBGH/rBST.

Read the labels in the store. If a label does not say "certified organic" or "rBGH/rBST free," there is a very good chance those cows were exposed and that milk is unsafe.

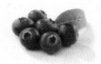

PART 4

Eating for Healing

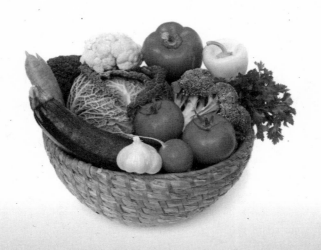

(a brief note for breast cancer survivors)

This short section primarily emphasizes the key principle that a diet and lifestyle to prevent cancer recurrence is in close concordance with the principles of its primary prevention. There are a few adjustments to be made by breast cancer survivors, but for the most part these recommendations will be familiar.

The major reason for creating a separate section here is that women who are being treated for cancer or who have completed treatment often wonder if the "rules have changed" for them. There seems to be a great uneasiness among cancer survivors, not being sure of how to decide which foods and supplements may help and which may actually harm. And doctors generally are not very helpful in advising in this area.

Though this chapter may seem repetitive, it is purposely included in order to reduce uncertainty and provide clarity to women after the diagnosis of cancer has already been made. And the really encouraging conclusion of the matter is this: your good choices really do make a difference for the better.

> **Large population studies of women with cancer have proven that food choices can enhance disease-free survival.**

Let's talk about what we know.

CHAPTER 15
Diet During Treatment and Preventing Recurrence

I will not attempt a comprehensive review of all the controversial recommendations around how to eat to optimize breast cancer treatment success or to prevent recurrence of the disease. Suffice it to say that the best minds in the field of integrative oncology recommend a diet during treatment that would look nearly identical to the risk reduction diet I have outlined already.

Soy Foods for Survivors

A couple of points to re-emphasize here are important. It is too early to give definitive recommendations on soy foods and estrogen-receptor-positive tumor recurrence. There were significant concerns about soy interfering with tamoxifen treatment, but the latest data actually showed benefit for women eating the highest amounts of soy protein.

Data are still being gathered, so if you choose to eat soy, stay with whole foods instead of soy protein extracts. Small to moderate amounts of whole soy foods (such as edamame or tofu) would be acceptable and perhaps even beneficial because of their flavonoid content.

Others would say this presents an unknown level of risk in possibly stimulating the tumor receptors and promoting growth. That would more likely be the case for concentrated soy protein products such as shakes, drink mixes and processed foods, but because of the uncertainty,

I must leave it to your personal taste preference. We simply don't know which way the data will go on this.

Continuing Protection from the "Broccoli Gang"

I also place a special emphasis on cruciferous vegetables because of their great value against estrogen-receptor-positive tumors. Indole-3-carbinol effects a change in estrogen metabolism to make tumor promotion less likely, and the other anticancer compounds in these vegetables are potent. Make a point of getting to know and love broccoli, cabbage, kale, cauliflower, brussel sprouts, bok choy and their family (reread Chapter 5, Cruciferous Vegetables for more detail on these foods).

Even More Caution about Trans-Fats and Hormones in Milk

Breast cancer survivors should be especially careful to avoid any dairy products that are from cows treated with growth hormone (RBGH or BST); these products carry the risk of unusual levels of a hormone called insulin-like growth factor (IGF) in the milk, which could be a tumor promoter.

Though this was outlined in some detail in the previous chapter, it is worth repeating here: Breast cancer survivors need to be very careful about avoiding trans-fats. Be a label reader and stay clear of foods with partially hydrogenated or hydrogenated oils.

Special Anticancer Additions to the Diet

Now for a discussion of some good things to eat in addition to the basic anti-inflammatory diet as outlined in the first chapter. Some mushrooms are worth getting to know and love if you have not already. The shiitake mushroom has been studied for decades and has known anti-cancer properties. Ideally, have at least one weekly serving.

> **Mushrooms must be cooked; humans cannot absorb the benefits of raw mushrooms.**

Other medicinal mushrooms are best derived as supplements because many are difficult or impossible to eat. The maitake mushroom is one species with known anti-tumor properties that can be found in some specialty groceries, but is also found in extract form in health food stores. It may be blended with other mushroom extracts with potent medicinal properties as well. An excellent source for quality products is Paul Stamets' company, *Fungi Perfecti*. These are organically produced supplements from one of the world's authorities on medicinal mushrooms.

Though this is not a food that Americans often eat, astragalus has been used as a medical herb in Chinese cooking for generations. It has potent effects on enhancing immunity and can be safely used by any cancer survivor during or after treatment. This can be found most commonly as an extract in pill form in health food stores. If you are an adventurous cook and have a Chinese grocery nearby, you could buy astragalus root and use it for soup stock, removing the woody root before serving.

What about taking your multivitamin or antioxidants during chemotherapy treatments? This has provoked controversy among oncologists, and some still recommend not taking these during treatment. A recent review of multiple studies of thousands of patients in active cancer treatment drew the following conclusions: One, the majority of clinical trials show that antioxidants during chemotherapy reduced side effects and either had no effect or improved treatment outcome and survival; and two, there was no evidence that antioxidants worsened treatment outcome.[1, 2]

I feel safe in recommending that women in treatment continue a good quality multivitamin-antioxidant blend.

Let's Help Doctors Learn Too!

Unfortunately, *nutritional illiteracy* is still commonplace among doctors. I have been told by more than one cancer patient that when they asked their oncologist about diet during treatment, they were told simply, "Eat a balanced diet." Not as helpful as one might hope. My hope is that this short chapter gives you the foundation for a healthy diet during and after treatment that can add to an optimal outcome.

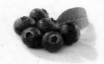

PART 5

Integrative Medicine— The Future of Health Care

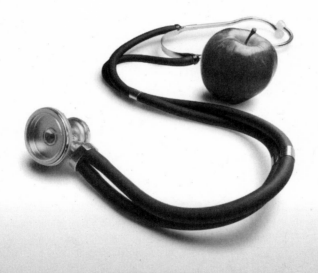

Having focused the entirety of this book so far on breast cancer risk reduction, I want to step back now and consider the health of the whole person. I believe that 100 percent of my cancer patients have said to me in these or similar words, "I want to do all I can to strengthen my entire system." That is an holistic look at human health—as a dynamic interplay between harmonized systems within an individual—and is the core approach of Integrative Medicine.

This section is written as if you had come to me in my office and asked the question, "What can I do to be healthier?" "How can I strengthen the system?" How do I make deposits into my health account?"

There are many perspectives in answering those questions. Let's explore a few of them together now.

CHAPTER 16
Eight Domains of Health for Prevention and Wellness

Interestingly, if you come to my medical office for a prevention and wellness appointment, much of the advice you will receive will be the same whether you are primarily interested in cancer prevention, heart disease prevention or healthy aging in general. There are numerous biochemical reasons for the broad applicability of my wellness recommendations.

These have to do with altering the concentration of stress hormones in the body, decreasing inflammation through food choices, minimizing toxic exposures, getting an adequate supply of antioxidants in the diet, and keeping blood and lymphatic flow open through regular physical activity. A biochemist or medical physiologist could go into great detail in all of those areas, but the longer I practice medicine and the more I read, the more amazed I am at the intricate complexity of the human organism, and how inadequate are any of our explanations on how interventions really change health on a cellular level.

Instead, as a practicing physician, I find metaphors and language that sounds more like poetry better at capturing why a single set of recommendations for health should have such a profound effect on so many different systems.

Much More like a Garden than a Machine

Let's think of human health as a vegetable garden. You'd like your garden to produce several different kinds of food (e.g. heart health, digestive health, mental health and feminine health), and you'd like to avoid the place being grown over by weeds (e.g. cancers), which choke out the other healthy plants. How to make all that happen?

Start with healthy soil, which means natural nutrients for the plants, just the right amount of water and avoiding chemical contaminants in your garden. Choose a place that gets plenty of sunlight, and also some shade late in the day to avoid overheating. Go for plant variety, since disease is more likely to take over a garden where only one crop is planted.

Put the seeds in the ground at the right time with respect to the seasons, the weather and the rhythms of nature. Once seeds are planted and watered, step back and trust the wisdom of the earth to bring them up at the right time; they do not thrive if you pull them up every day to check and see if they have roots yet. When the plants are up and growing, take some time every single day to tend the garden. That means pulling weeds, squashing pests by hand if necessary to protect your garden and even sweating and getting dirty from some hard work every day to keep the garden from being taken over by the natural threats to life on earth.

And then, when your prized plants produce their crops, don't just stand back and look; harvest the fruits of your labor, bring them in the kitchen and get "cookin'" with gratitude! You deserve to enjoy the good fruits of your labor year after year. And finally, no matter how proud you are of this year's garden, it won't feed you next year. Growing anything means you plant new seeds every spring.

Putting Good Gardening into Practice in the Body

I hope those metaphors prompt some thinking for you about how you care about the garden of your health and your body. You will probably discover other meanings even beyond those I do for myself, but I will share a few of my thoughts about the healthy lifestyle implied by the garden metaphor.

The components of a healthy "soil" for the human body consist of building blocks that are nutritional foods. For good health, the body requires constant replenishment with the purest and most complete building blocks available. Consuming plenty of water is the key to moving nutrients in and toxins out. A wide array of nutritional foods provides the building blocks for healthy cells, just like a gardener would till in large amounts of organic compost to make the soil hospitable for healthy plants.

Keep chemical contaminants out by eating organically grown foods whenever possible, and avoid exposing your cells to toxins that can cause mutations. Sunlight is important for humans quite literally, since this is the very best way to make vitamin D, a crucial hormone that regulates cell growth and immunity.

Then, remember to respect the rhythms of nature. When the sun goes down, it's time to slow down and rest; the plants in your garden are not made to be in the sun 24/7. Your body also needs quiet, shade and rest for a long uninterrupted time every 24-hour period.

Then there's the important balance between diligent work to protect your body's health and the joyful gratitude for how well the system works all by itself when you are just going about life. Yes, you've got to cultivate good habits of exercise, diet and toxin avoidance, and pull out the weeds of disease as they sprout, get regular checkups and screening tests, but don't be so health-obsessed that every day presents a set of serious decisions. Who wants to have dinner with someone who is talking about the biochemical benefits of their food for health?

Relax a bit after you've made healthy choices, and just enjoy life without anxiety. And do some fun things with that healthy body! Instead of using health as an end in itself, find ways to enjoy the fruits of your efforts: Take a dance class; go on a picnic or a hike on a weekend morning; get up and watch a sunrise; take a canoe trip; play tennis; celebrate your healthy body with a massage. Use your own imagination and creativity!

A Reason to be Healthy

Another key concept for me is that one needs some purpose for living. Otherwise, why be healthy? A long life is worth living for people with a clear sense of purpose, but without that purpose I find that people are not very motivated to make changes for better health. Without a sense of mission and purpose, why not just spend your time enjoying temporal pleasures of food, drink and adventure? But a person with a compelling mission will want to stay healthy in order to move toward a passion-producing goal.

Wellness in All Areas

When I see patients in my office for wellness consults, I generally cover recommendations in eight distinct but overlapping areas. These are:
- conventional medicine,
- nutritional medicine,
- herbs and dietary supplements,
- mind-body medicine,
- physical activity and bodywork,
- energy medicine,
- spirituality and relationships, and
- environment.

Conventional Medicine

Wellness recommendations from a conventional medical perspective depend on your age, gender and other demographic factors. These include such recommendations as mammograms, colonoscopy, stool hemoccult testing and bone density screening. You can actually find customized scientific recommendations based on your age and gender at *http://epss.ahrq.gov/ePSS/search.jsp.* This website has a searchable database of specific recommendations from the U.S. Preventive Services Task Force. Type in your age, gender and other information, then get details on the evidence-based recommendations for your personal situation.

Nutritional Medicine

As you might suspect after reading thus far, *nutritional medicine* forms much of the foundation for my prevention and wellness recommendations for anyone. The anti-inflammatory diet is so broadly applicable that it makes it into the written recommendations for almost all of my patients. If you are still uncertain what this entails, see Andrew Weil's link to the anti-inflammatory food pyramid at *http://www.drweil.com/* This diet could just as well be called the anticancer diet or the healthy aging diet.

Herbs and Dietary Supplements

There are some herbs and dietary supplements that make it regularly into my prevention recommendations also. Fish oil (omega-3 fatty acids, especially concentrated DHA and EPA) has broad preventive potential. Persons who do not regularly eat garlic could benefit from a daily supplement, and I often tell patients if they are not eating at least one clove of fresh garlic daily, to take a garlic extract in pill form.

A daily multivitamin is also important, especially for its antioxidant contents: Vitamin C, vitamin A as natural carotenoids, vitamin E as natural tocopherols, and selenium are all key components of a daily multivitamin, taken as a sort of "insurance" policy for the days we don't eat "perfectly." Vitamin D gets a special emphasis as well. Not only for bone health, vitamin D deficiencies are common and probably contribute to many of the chronic diseases we experience, including depression, diabetes, heart disease, auto-immune diseases and some cancers.

I recommend a daily maintenance dose of 1,000 IU of vitamin D3 for all patients over the age of 12, and 400 IU for children. If your level has been tested and found to be low (below 32 ng/mL), increase your intake up to 4,000 IU per day, then retest before going back to a maintenance level of 1,000 IU.

Mind-Body Medicine

Mind-body medicine gets scarcely a mention in conventional medical circles as a prevention strategy, but I view it as an indispensable foundation. The simplest and most broadly applicable of these practices is conscious breath work. Two five-minute or 10-minute breathing breaks in the middle of a busy day can shift your body out of stress responses and into cellular healing. There are many good references on breathing exercises; refer to the writings of Deepak Chopra (*Grow Younger, Live Longer*) and Andrew Weil (*Eight Weeks to Optimum Health*) for detailed examples of healthy breathing practices.

To start, I recommend simply using breath observation:

Sit quietly in one place, legs uncrossed, arms comfortably in the lap. Let the eyes close, and allow your attention to be completely given to the breath moving in and out, in and out. The mind will wander, no doubt about it, and when it does, don't be critical of yourself, just gently bring your attention back to the breath.

At first this may be frustrating, but with daily practice, you will feel the benefits by being calmer, clearer in thinking and less stressed. Not only does this make for a better day, it actually protects your body and your immune system.

Regular Physical Activity

There is no prescription I can write that has as many and as far-reaching effects as exercise and *regular physical activity*: better bone health, less depression, weight control, decreased risk of diabetes, decreased risk of heart disease and many cancers. No pill in any drugstore can do all that for you. Yet this is one of the least common health practices for most of the American population. Clearly there is a disconnect between what we know (You already knew the importance of exercise before reading this paragraph, right?) and taking action on what we know.

It seems intuitive, and has also been shown by well researched studies, that health-related activities such as exercise are driven by the individual mind seeking a balance of pain and pleasure, gain and loss. Anytime you are asked to change in some way, there is both gain and loss at stake.

As a way to demonstrate this, use this short exercise:

Consider your current habitual exercise pattern, specifically the question, how many days in the past week did you do any aerobic exercise for at least 30 minutes? And was this past week typical of your past month, past year? Or was it the exception?

Take a moment to honestly appraise yourself and your exercise habits based on this question. Consider your own data without either self-criticism or self-congratulation. Facts are facts, and you are just allowing your mind to focus on the honest facts.

Now take a moment to sit quietly, uncross the legs, place your hands comfortably in your lap, and ask the question, "If I continue this pattern for the rest of my life, what are the benefits to me, and what are the costs to me?"

For example, if you have been sedentary, the benefits of continuing that pattern are that you won't have any expense of joining the gym or buying new running shoes; you may be able to sleep longer in the morning and be able to stay cool and comfortable in your house. And the costs to consider of staying sedentary would be increasing your chances of heart disease, cancer, diabetes, obesity and depression.

Does the pain of those costs outweigh the pleasure of the benefits? If not, how can you make the pain of the costs seem more real, rather than an abstract possibility in an imagined future?

Now flip the imaginary scenario around. Picture yourself getting regular physical activity. One easy way to do this is to remember a time when you were exercising regularly and recall how it felt. Bring those feelings into the present, and into the imagined future. Is there a sense of pride and accomplishment? Can you vividly see in your mind's eye a fit and toned body?

Perhaps allow yourself to picture even the shared camaraderie of working out or playing a sport with others of your age and interests. And just like picturing the pain and pleasure of staying sedentary, take a few moments in quiet reflection to consider the costs and benefits of regular physical activity.

This exercise brings into the area of conscious control a process that is going on in the subconscious mind daily. Our minds are always weighing the cost/benefit ratio of any behavior we are considering, especially those that involve a radical change in habits. Bringing that weighing and comparison process into the light of consciousness allows you to be in control of the decision, rather than letting your life be driven by old conditioning and habits that may not serve you well.

I sincerely hope that such a process will lead you into a clarifying insight about your own exercise choices, and that you will find it easier to choose regular physical activity, a lifesaving (lifetime) habit!

Bodywork

Alongside regular physical activity, I recommend some attention to *bodywork* as a good preventive health habit. Regular therapeutic massage is a great stress reducer, balances muscles and soft tissue, prevents pain, promotes better sleep and improves lymphatic flow. Other special types of massage and bodywork include such fields as structural integration and may be helpful for those with postural imbalances. If you choose regular chiropractic work as a health promotion strategy, I recommend you work with a chiropractor who minimizes the use of X-rays; any use of X-rays adds slightly to risk of cancer. They should not be used unless necessary.

If you are fortunate enough to live in a community with an osteopathic physician (D.O.) who practices traditional osteopathic manipulation, this is a very beneficial practice for addressing imbalances in muscle and soft tissue. Unfortunately, there are very few Doctors of Osteopathy who still practice this medical art.

Energy Medicine

From ancient times to now, cultures around the world have recognized that the human body is penetrated by and surrounded with an invisible energy field. Various systems of energy healing, or *energy medicine*, have attempted to address this energy both to prevent and treat disease.

The ancient medicine of India, Ayurveda, recognized the existence of *chakras*, energy centers in the body, which served as portals for energy moving in and out of the body. The invisible energy in this system of Ayurveda is called *Prana*.

Traditional Chinese medicine uses acupuncture to enhance the flow of *Qi* (chee) along invisible energy meridians that carry health messages throughout the body; the ancient Chinese practice of *Qigong* (chee gung) also works with Qi in order to build it up and improve its flow in the body.

> **Qigong was my first introduction personally to the idea of energy medicine, when I ran across a magazine article describing its use years ago. I began practicing Qigong from books and video instruction. I received subsequent teaching from masters like Roger Jahnke, and have since seen its power at work in individuals and classes.**

Modern variations on these ancient energy practices include Healing Touch and Reiki among others. These are different schools of energy healing, which are aimed at assessing and manipulating the body's energy fields in order to provide physical comfort and enhance health. To some these practices may sound unscientific and esoteric. I have personally seen them benefit many people, and recommend them regularly as ways to enhance health and augment other approaches to the treatment of disease.

Spirituality and Relationships

The area of *spirituality* and *relationships* is a very important domain to consider in health promotion and prevention of disease. To be a whole person means having a sense of meaning and purpose in life—some connection to something bigger than oneself—and an appreciation of invisible transcendent qualities of our existence like beauty, truth, fairness, wonder and love.

Being a whole person means not only having a sense that those qualities exist; but also a sense that somehow one's daily activities of work, vocation or hobbies, for example, bring one into closer alignment with those values. That's what I mean by spirituality. This is often connected with some organized religion or philosophy, but not necessarily so.

Closely tied to that concept of spirituality is the health domain of relationships. People in isolation from other people are missing a key part of what it means to be human. Most of the significance of our lives comes in the context of relationships: Who supports us, and whom do we support? With whom do we share a sense of love and fondness? Are there mentoring relationships in your life, either giving or receiving?

If for some reason relationships are missing or weak, I recommend to my patients to find more ways to connect, to spend time with people who make them feel more alive and connected. This again makes intuitive sense, but has also been shown to be associated with more positive health outcomes and longevity.

Environment

The final domain of preventive health I cover with patients is that of *environment*. You have already heard from me the importance of eating organically when possible, and keeping other toxins out of the body. One more toxin exposure to emphasize here is that of our drinking and bathing water. As we've discussed, chlorination is a very useful process for ridding municipal drinking water of disease-causing microbes, and this is one major advance in public health in the past century.

But chlorine is also a potent toxin and can add to risk of cancers. It combines with leftover organic molecules in the water system, such as breakdown of vegetation, and makes compounds such as trihalomethanes, known carcinogens. These can be ingested in drinking water and also inhaled and absorbed through the skin, for example, while taking a hot shower.

For this reason, I strongly recommend a point-of-use drinking water filter to use at your tap in the home: Buy a filter certified to remove chlorine at the very least. There are commercially available filters for the showerhead as well, designed to remove chlorine and other chemicals from the hot water and steam you run over your skin and breathe. Look for a filter certified by NSF, the National Sanitation Foundation.

And to avoid environmental toxins in food, use the "Dirty Dozen" list from the Environmental Working Group to choose organics without breaking your budget. Even if you make a commitment to choose organics only for the top 10 contaminated foods, you reduce your toxic load by perhaps 90 percent and still don't have to buy all of your groceries organically. See *http://www.FoodNews.org* for this useful guide.

Begin and End With Gratitude

While I view food and nutrition as the single most important area that you can control for breast cancer risk reduction, I hope you have a sense now that the process of adding to your health and wellness encompasses a wide array of practices and habits: from spirituality to stress reduction to exercise and more. It's really about creating balance in life, a sense of ease and completeness, fully alive and fully connected for as long as you live.

And that thought leads me directly to one concluding concept: gratitude. The more you build on these foundational principles, the more you will find reason to pause with gratitude every day. Gratitude for the gift of life, for the gifts of food, breath, movement and relationships is a way to keep the heart open and young. Gratitude for the gifts you have already received opens the possibility of more gifts arriving daily, whereas a person without gratitude will not be open to receiving more.

Why would the architect of the universe want to give more gifts to someone who was not thankful for what they already had? Pause, then, for gratitude when you awake in the morning, when you step outside and see the sunlight, when you sit down to a meal, and when you lie down at night after a busy day. Gratitude alone can change your life.

Epilogue:
Reflections on the Mission

At the outset of creating this book, my reasons for writing were very clear and simple.

> **Most women did not know that they could make choices every day that would decrease their chance of ever having breast cancer.**

Despite all of the reliable and powerful information I could access as a professional about the nutritional approaches to breast cancer risk reduction, it appeared to me in my patient encounters and in observations of public life that there was a critical shortage of such information where it counted the most. Women were going about their daily lives with a sense of fatalism, just hoping they were lucky enough to avoid breast cancer, often living in fear day after day.

This helpless fear unfortunately has been in part driven by a medical establishment that is not only focused more on treatment than on prevention, but is also functionally illiterate in nutrition.

And individual doctors are really not to blame. They are doing their jobs as well as they can with the training they have had. Their training is in treatment of disease much more so than its prevention, and nutritional medicine is still a marginal topic in medical school curricula. It takes more than a little effort for a practicing physician to become knowledgeable enough about nutrition to make solid recommendations.

The widespread application of this sort of knowledge to medical practice may have to wait for a whole new generation of physicians to come along, while women continue to wait in fear for the occurrence of breast cancer or in the hope they are lucky enough to dodge it.

But why wait?

> **You now have enough practical information
> to take control of your health future.**

The suggestions given in this book are based on reliable science and will considerably decrease your risk of breast cancer. And I believe this is achievable thanks to a dietary plan and lifestyle choices that can be fulfilling, satisfying, tasty and fun!

It's a good time to reiterate that any risk reduction plan such as the one outlined here does not guarantee any outcome. Any individual following these recommendations perfectly still could be diagnosed with breast cancer. It is just statistically much less likely to happen. The American Institute for Cancer Research estimated this year that 38 percent of the expected number of breast cancer cases in the U.S. could be prevented by diet, physical activity and weight control. With 194,000 new breast cancer cases diagnosed yearly in the U.S., that 38 percent amounts to more than 73,000 people each year who do not have to hear that really bad news from a doctor when the biopsy report comes in.

And every one of those 73,000 was once a little toddler, like Dianne's granddaughter who will never know her. Every one of those 73,000 was at one time a beautiful teenage girl wondering what she could wear to look her best. Every one of those 73,000 can someday be a music teacher, or a dancer, or an executive, a researcher, writer, doctor, mother, grandmother, or a retired traveler enjoying a long, rewarding life of giving and receiving. This is the number that keeps me up late at night working to get the word out!

I know those people personally. I know their sisters, mothers, children and friends. I have seen what breast cancer can do to women and their families and friends. *It doesn't have to happen so often.* It will clearly take more than one book to make the changes that are needed, but it is my sincere hope that this book and its message can make it into the hands of millions of women, who can then begin making these changes to save lives.

Can You Help Spread the Word?

On a personal note, I have found as a physician and educator for the past 25 years that practical and reliable information such as that found in this book is in woefully short supply for public consumption. My wife and I teach health classes and seminars together, and we find that people are overwhelmingly grateful to receive clear and empowering information.

The bookstores, media outlets, and airwaves are jammed with sensational headlines and diet plans that remain popular until the next fad comes along. And in that atmosphere where much of the information may as well be audio and visual static, more women daily continue to receive bad news from a biopsy. My hope is that a number of women each day—real names and faces with families and children and houses and gardens—will be plucked out of that "bad news" group and never know that they might have been in it.

I have tried to "do the math" and answer the question of how many books will have to get into people's hands in order statistically to save one life. That math problem has stumped me, but I know with certainty that the answer is "more will make a bigger difference and save more lives." If you find the information in this book to be useful and hopeful for you, please help the mission by purchasing a copy for a friend as well.

Don't wait for a doctor to tell you. Start now. And spread the word. Someone you know needs to know this . . . Today. Today is a gift; share the gift of empowerment with someone today, and tell her that her choices really do make a difference. I hope that will bring a smile to someone's face. It certainly will to mine.

Robert Pendergrast, MD

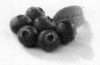

Appendix 1:
Breast Health Action Plan

This simple worksheet will help you through the steps it will take to implement the principles in this book.

I am including this action plan worksheet because I assume you are ready to take some action by the time you have reached this point in the book. But I also encourage you to be gentle with yourself and not demand radical changes in too many areas at once if that feels too difficult. Make changes that are realistic, measurable, and *that you feel certain you can achieve* in three week increments—even just one. That is, start with three weeks of success—even a single small success. Mark and celebrate that success at the end of the three weeks and then look at the worksheet again for additional steps you can take.

For that reason, I suggest you photocopy the worksheet pages so they can be used over again when you make additional healthy changes in your life. These worksheets can also be downloaded from the website, *http://www.breasthealthplan.com*

Instructions:

On the line for each category, each line having a series of numbers indicating grades from zero to 10, place the letters N (for Now) and I (for Ideal) at the numbers representing your own self-assessment of your health behavior. For example, on the line marked *cruciferous vegetables,* you would place the letter "N" (Now) at a number indicating how you see yourself NOW on cruciferous vegetables intake for cancer prevention, zero being the worst, and 10 being the best. Then place the letter "I" (Ideal) at the number that represents your short term goal for that intake during the next three weeks.

Below the line, you will find a blank line to answer the questions: "how much; how often; by when?" Your answers to those questions will give you a specific goal which you can measure for self-assessment at the end of three weeks. For example, you might say, "I will eat at least one half cup serving of a cruciferous vegetable every other day, starting tomorrow, January 25." It must be specific and measurable. An answer like "I will eat more broccoli in the next three weeks" does not count.

Now take each of these areas, grade your current state, your three week goal, and write your measurable action plan.

1. Colorful Diet

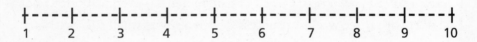

Mark **N** for "Now," and **I** for "Ideal goal" in the next three weeks. My measurable, specific goal for the next three weeks is:

_____

2. Exercise

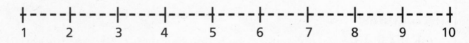

Mark **N** for "Now," and **I** for "Ideal goal" in the next three weeks. My measurable, specific goal for the next three weeks is:

_____

3. Environmental Toxins

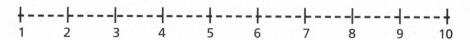

Mark **N** for "Now," and **I** for "Ideal goal" in the next three weeks.
My measurable, specific goal for the next three weeks is:

_____

4. Whole Soy Foods

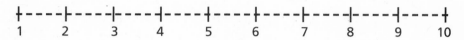

Mark **N** for "Now," and **I** for "Ideal goal" in the next three weeks.
My measurable, specific goal for the next three weeks is:

_____

5. Cruciferous Vegetables

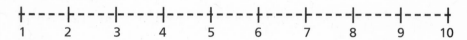

Mark **N** for "Now," and **I** for "Ideal goal" in the next three weeks.
My measurable, specific goal for the next three weeks is:

_____

6. High Omega-3 Fish

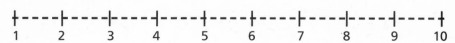

Mark **N** for "Now," and **I** for "Ideal goal" in the next three weeks.
My measurable, specific goal for the next three weeks is:

_____

7. Flax Seed

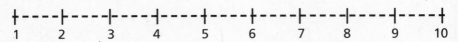

Mark **N** for "Now," and **I** for "Ideal goal" in the next three weeks.
My measurable, specific goal for the next three weeks is:

_____

8. Healing Spices

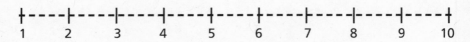

Mark **N** for "Now," and **I** for "Ideal goal" in the next three weeks.
My measurable, specific goal for the next three weeks is:

_____

9. Healthy Mushrooms

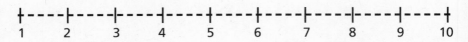

Mark **N** for "Now," and **I** for "Ideal goal" in the next three weeks.
My measurable, specific goal for the next three weeks is:

_____

10. Berries

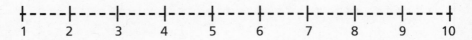

Mark **N** for "Now," and **I** for "Ideal goal" in the next three weeks.
My measurable, specific goal for the next three weeks is:

_____

11. Green Leafy Vegetables

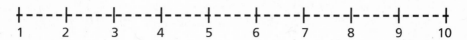

Mark **N** for "Now," and **I** for "Ideal goal" in the next three weeks.

My measurable, specific goal for the next three weeks is:

---

12. Tea

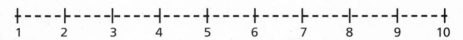

Mark **N** for "Now," and **I** for "Ideal goal" in the next three weeks.

My measurable, specific goal for the next three weeks is:

---

13. Avoiding Toxic Doses of Alcohol and Grilled Meat

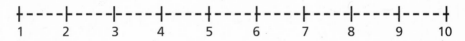

Mark **N** for "Now," and **I** for "Ideal goal" in the next three weeks.

My measurable, specific goal for the next three weeks is:

---

14. Avoiding Environmental Toxins Such as Trans-Fats, Hormones in Milk and PCB's

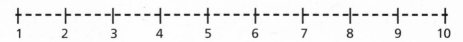

Mark **N** for "Now," and **I** for "Ideal goal" in the next three weeks.

My measurable, specific goal for the next three weeks is:

Congratulations on taking the time to create changes that can make a big difference in your health!

And one final action step, one that I think you will enjoy. Thinking again of the metaphor of your health as a garden (see Chapter 16, Eight Domains of Health for Prevention and Wellness), review those eight areas of health and wellness and consider which one or two you could cultivate more to yield a fruitful harvest of health in your life. Perhaps it would be making some stress reduction practice such as meditation or conscious breathing a habit, or discovering some new meaning or purpose in your life such as a hobby or some volunteer work. Whatever you choose, be assured that energy invested in the garden of your health will be multiplied in future vitality and well being.

Appendix 2: Resources

Books

Katz, R., Edelson, M. *The Cancer Fighting Kitchen: Nourishing, Big-Flavor Recipes for Cancer Treatment and Recovery.* **Berkeley: Celestial Arts, 2009.**
This beautifully illustrated cookbook is also filled with good information on how to eat for prevention, and has sections of special recommendations on how to eat during different stages of cancer treatment.

Dr. Susan Love's Breast Book, 4th edition. **Cambridge: Da Capo Press, 2005.**
Written by a breast surgeon, this is the most comprehensive book on breast health for non-medical audiences. It thoroughly covers anatomy, development of the breast over the lifespan, explanations of breast diseases and different types of tumors, and how surgery and medical therapy are used in treating breast cancer.

Block, K., MD. *Life Over Cancer: the Block Center Program for Integrative Cancer Treatment.* **Bantam Books, 2009.**
This is a written blueprint of how the Block Cancer Center in Evanston Illinois approaches cancer treatments in an integrative fashion. Dr. Block is an oncologist and a recognized leader in the Society for Integrative Oncology. Here you will find a truly effective and science-based combination of conventional cancer treatments and natural remedies that enhance treatment.

**Abrams, D., and Weil, A., eds. *Integrative Oncology.*
Oxford University Press, 2009.**
A scholarly edition in the Oxford University Press' Weil Integrative Medicine Library, this is a collaboration between Dr. Abrams, an oncologist at San Francisco General Hospital, and Dr. Weil, the leading innovator in bringing natural medicine into the mainstream. Many other experts in the field contributed to this textbook. It is written as a medical reference volume for physicians who wish to bring Integrative Medicine to Oncology.

**Weil, A., MD. *Eating Well for Optimum Health.*
HarperCollins, 2000.**
Dr. Weil's classic volume on the power of good food for the prevention and treatment of disease, no home should be without it.

**Weil, A., MD. *Healthy Aging: a Lifelong Guide to Your Well-Being.*
Random House, 2005.**
In a reassuring and meticulously well-thought book, Dr. Weil crafts a response to "anti-aging" medicine. He shows how much better it is to acknowledge growing older as a potential for growth and change, while using natural medicine and wellness as the way to stay healthy and vibrant far into old age.

**Jahnke, R., OMD. *The Healer Within.*
HarperCollins, 1997.**
Drawing on years of practice and teaching of Chinese Medicine, Qigong (chee-kung) and Tai-chi, Dr. Jahnke presents a simple set of gentle exercises and breathing techniques which unlock the inner pharmacy, or as he says "the most profound medicine." Illustrated and easy to follow, it is a treasure of self-applied healing methods.

Carson, Rachel. *Silent Spring: 40th Anniversary Edition.* Mariner Books, 2002.

One of the most influential writers of the 20th century, this pivotal work in 1962 first alerted the American public of the dangers to our health and to our planet of chemical based agriculture. Her notion that we could actually destroy the earth and ourselves in the process was new and radical thinking then, and it is no less important today.

Internet Resources

http://www.holistic-medicine-md.com
Dr. Pendergrast's free internet resource for the best in holistic medicine recommendations for prevention and wellness. It includes a link to sign up for *Real Foods That Heal,* his periodic e-zine sent to subscribers.

http://www.aikenaugustaholistichealth.com
For those in the southeastern US, Dr. Pendergrast's Integrative Medicine practice is within one day's driving distance. He welcomes consults of all ages by appointment.

http://integrativemedicine.arizona.edu/
The Center for Integrative Medicine at the University of Arizona was founded by Dr. Andrew Weil. Dr. Pendergrast is a graduate of the program and continues to be active in their education programs. One can find a graduate of the program by using the "practitioner finder" on the website, and easily locate an Integrative Medicine practitioner in cities all over the United States and several other countries.

http://www.nutritionandhealthconf.org/

The premier educational event of its kind; physicians, registered dietitians and other professionals gather yearly to learn the most updated cutting edge information on nutrition and health.

http://www.blockmd.com/

For 30 years, Keith Block M.D. has directed the most comprehensive integrative cancer center in the United States. Located in Evanston, Illinois, they accept referrals from anywhere.

http://www.foodnews.org/

The shopper's guide to pesticides. Want to eat organically but not spend so much? This is the definitive guide to how to avoid the most heavily pesticide laden foods, and how choosing the "cleanest" produce items from conventional agriculture can be safe and more economical.

http://www.montereybayaquarium.org/cr/seafoodwatch.aspx

This is a practically organized guide to buying and choosing seafood in the market or in restaurants. You will find which fish are highest in healthy omega-3 fats and which are harvested from sustainable fisheries for the health of the oceans and our planet.

End Notes

Introduction

1. This is speaking of conventional allopathic medical schools where MD's start their careers. Naturopathic schools have a long history of emphasizing both nutrition and preventive medicine.

2. Preamble to the Constitution of the World Health Organization as adopted by the International Health Conference, New York, 19-22 June, 1946; signed on 22 July, 1946, by the representatives of 61 States (Official Records of the World Health Organization, no. 2, p. 100) and entered into force on 7 April, 1948.

Chapter 1

1. World Cancer Research Fund / American Institute for Cancer Research. "Food, Nutrition, Physical Activity, and the Prevention of Cancer: a Global Perspective." Washington DC: AICR (2007).

2. Smith-Warner, S., et al. "Intake of Fruits and Vegetables and Risk of Breast Cancer: a pooled analysis of cohort studies." *JAMA* (2001):285; 769-776.

3. Pollan, Michael. *In Defense of Food: An Eater's Manifesto.* Penguin Press, 2008.

4. Heber D., with Bowermann, S. *What Color is Your Diet? The Seven Colors of Health* (New York: HarperCollins, 2001).

5. Trichopoulou, A. "Consumption of Olive Oil and Specific Food Groups in Relation to Breast Cancer Risk in Greece." *Journal of the National Cancer Institute* (1995, January 18): Vol. 87, No. 2, 110-116.

6. Chajes, V., et al. "Association between serum trans-monounsaturated fatty acids and breast cancer risk in the E3N-EPIC Study." *American Journal of Epidemiology* (2008, Jun 1): 167(11)1312-20.

7. Liu, S., Manson, J.E., Buring, J.E., et al. Relation between a diet with a high glycemic load and plasma concentrations of high-sensitivity C-reactive protein in middle-aged women." *Am J Clin Nutr* (2002):75, 492-8.

8. Thun, M.J., Henley, S.J., Gansler, T. "Inflammation and cancer: an epidemiological perspective." *Novartis Found Symp* (2004):256,6-21.

9. For more details on the glycemic index, see the work of Dr. Jennie Brand-Miller at the University of Sydney, at *www.glycemicindex.com*.

Chapter 2

1. Dallal, C.M., et al. "Long-term recreational physical activity and risk of invasive and in situ breast cancer: the California teachers study." *Archives of Internal Medicine* (2007, Feb 26):167(4) 408-15.

2. Blair, S.N., Connelly, J.C. "How much physical activity should we do?" *Res Q Exerc Sport* (1996):67(2) 193-205.

Chapter 3

1. Cardis E., et al. "Estimates of the Cancer Burden in Europe from Radioactive Fallout from the Chernobyl Accident." *Int. J. Cancer:* (2006):119, 1224–1235.

2. See the American Cancer Society's information at *http://www.cancer.org* for example.

3. Chisato Nagata, et al. and Shoichiro Tsugane Research Group for the Development and Evaluation of Cancer Prevention Strategies in Japan. "Tobacco Smoking and Breast Cancer Risk: An Evaluation Based on a Systematic Review of Epidemiological Evidence among the Japanese Population." *Japanese Journal of Clinical Oncology.* 2006(36): 387-394.

4. This information is publicly available through such online resources as the Seafood Selector page from the Environmental Defense Fund, at *http://www.edf.org*.

5. National Cancer Institute data at *http://www.cancer.gov/cancertopics/fact-sheet/Risk/heterocyclic-amines*.

6. Melnick R, et al. "Trihalomethanes and Other Environmental Factors That Contribute to Colorectal Cancer." *Environmental Health Perspectives* (1994): Volume 102, Number 6-7, June-July.

7. For information on how to choose organic foods most cost-effectively by avoiding only the most contaminated foods on the market, and about plastics and other hormone disruptors in the environment, see the Internet resources of the Environmental Working Group (*http://www.foodnews.org/* and *http://www.ewg.org/health*).

Chapter 4

1. Limer, J., Speirs, V. "Phyto-oestrogens and Breast Cancer Chemoprevention." *Breast Cancer Res* (2004): 6:119-127.

2. Li-Qian Qin et al. "Soyfood intake in the prevention of breast cancer risk in women: a meta-analysis of observational epidemiologic studies." *J Nutri Sci Vitaminol*, 52, 428-436, 2006.

3. Guha, N., et al. "Soy isoflavones and risk of cancer recurrence in a cohort of breast cancer survivors: the Life After Cancer Epidemiology study." *Breast Cancer Res Treat.* (2009 Nov): 118(2):395-405.

Chapter 5

1. Fink, B. N., Steck, S.E., Wolff, M.S., Britton, J.A., Kabat, G.C., Schroeder, J.C., Teitelbaum, S.L., Neugut, A.I., and Gammon, M.D. 2007. "Dietary flavonoid intake and breast cancer risk among women on Long Island." *Am J Epidemiol.* 2007, Mar 1; 165(5):514-23.

Chapter 6

1. Tapiero, H., Guyen, Ba, G., Couvreur, P., Tew, K.D. "Polyunsaturated fatty acids (PUFA) and eicosanoids in human health and pathologies." *Biomed Pharmacother* (2002): 56, 215–222.

2. Please refer to the Seafood Selector at the Environmental Defense Fund's website, *http://www.edf.org/home.cfm* for more information on fish choices that are good for you and the planet.

Chapter 8

1. Verma, S. P., Salamone, E., and Goldin, B. "Curcumin and Genistein, Plant Natural Products Show Synergistic Inhibitory Effects on the Growth of Human Breast Cancer MCF-7 Cells Induced by Estrogenic Pesticides." *Biochemical and Biophysical Research Communications* (1997): 233, 692–696.

2. Grzanna, R., et al. "Ginger extract inhibits beta-amyloid peptide-induced cytokine and chemokine expression in cultured THP-1 monocytes." *Journal of Alternative & Complementary Medicine* (2004, Dec): 10(6) 1009-13.

3. Choi, J.A., et al. "Induction of cell cycle arrest and apoptosis in human breast cancer cells by quercitin." *International Journal of Oncology* (2001, Oct): 19(4) 837-44.

Chapter 9

1. Grube, B., et al. "White Button Mushroom Phytochemicals Inhibit Aromatase Activity and Breast Cancer Cell Proliferation." *J. Nutr.* (2001): 131, 3288–3293.

2. Jiang, J., et al. "Ganoderma lucidum suppresses growth of breast cancer cells through the inhibition of Akt/NF-kappaB signaling." *Nutrition and Cancer* (2004): 49(2) 209-16.

3. Lu, Q.Y., et al. "Ganoderma lucidum spore extract inhibits endothelial and breast cancer cells in vitro." *Oncology Reports* (2004): 12(3) 659-62.

4. Oikawa, S., et al. "Radical production and DNA damage induced by carcinogenic 4-hydrazinobenzoic acid, an ingredient of mushroom Agaricus bisporus." *Free Radic Res.* (2006 Jan);40(1):31-9.

Chapter 10

1. Olsson, M., et al. "Antioxidant levels and inhibition of cancer cell proliferation in vitro by extracts from organically and conventionally cultivated strawberries." *Journal of Agricultural & Food Chemistry* (2006): 54(4)1248-55.
2. Zhang, C.X. "Greater vegetable and fruit intake is associated with a lower risk of breast cancer among Chinese women." *International Journal of Cancer* (2009): 125(1)181-8.

3. See the *Shopper's Guide to Pesticides* published by the Environmental Working Group at *http://www.foodnews.org/*.

Chapter 11

1. Zhang, S., et al. "Dietary carotenoids and vitamins A, C, and E and risk of breast cancer." *Journal of the National Cancer Institute* (1999, Mar. 17): 91(6) 547-56.

2. Zhang, S., et al. Plasma Folate, Vitamin B6, Vitamin B12, Homocysteine, and Risk of Breast Cancer." *Journal of the National Cancer Institute* (2003, Mar. 5): 95(5) 373-80.

Chapter 12

1. Jin-Rong Zhou, Linglin Li, and Weijun Pan. "Dietary soy and tea combinations for prevention of breast and prostate cancers by targeting metabolic syndrome elements in mice." *Am J Clin Nutr* (2007): 86(suppl) 882S–8S.

Chapter 13

1. Kris-Etherton, P. et al. AHA Science Advisory: Lyon Diet Heart Study. "Benefits of a Mediterranean-style, National Cholesterol Education Program/American Heart Association Step I Dietary Pattern on Cardiovascular Disease." *Circulation*. (2001 Apr 3); 103(13): 1823-5.

2. The reduction in heart disease risk from moderate alcohol use is true for the population on average, but individual risk may go up or down depending

on one's genetic makeup, specifically the Apo-E gene. Roughly 20% of the population has an Apo-E 4 allele which makes cholesterol numbers get worse with moderate alcohol use.

3. World Cancer Research Fund /American Institute for Cancer Research. "Food, Nutrition, Physical Activity, and the Prevention of Cancer: a Global Perspective." (Washington DC: AICR, 2007).

4. Harvard Nutrition Source, *http://www.hsph.harvard.edu/nutrition-source/what-should-you-eat/alcohol-full-story/index.html.*

5. Wei Zheng et al. "Sulfotransferase 1A1 Polymorphism, Endogenous Estrogen Exposure, Well Done Meat Intake, and Breast Cancer Risk." *Cancer Epidemiology, Biomarkers and Prevention.* (February 2001): 10:89.

6. Wei Zheng et al. "Well Done Meat Intake and the Risk of Breast Cancer." *Journal of the National Cancer Institute,* (1998):90:1724-9.

Chapter 15

1. Block, K., Koch, A., Mead, M., Tothy, P., Newman, R., and Gyllenhaal, C. "Efficacy of Adjuvant Antioxidants and Cancer Chemotherapy: A Systematic Review of the Evidence from Randomized Controlled Trials." *Cancer Treat Rev* (2007, Aug.): 33(5) 407-18.

2. Block, K., Koch, A., Mead, M., Tothy, P., Newman, R., and Gyllenhaal, "Impact of Antioxidant Supplementation on Chemotherapeutic Toxicity: A Systematic Review Of The Evidence from Randomized Controlled Trials." *Int J Cancer* (2008, Sep. 15): 123(6)1227-39.

References

American Botanical Council. 1999. "Flax: Ancient Herb and Modern Medicine." (*HerbalGram*; 45:51-57).

American Cancer Society. 2008. "Breast Cancer Facts & Figures 2007-2008." (Atlanta: American Cancer Society, Inc.).

Adachi, K., et al. 1987. "Potentiation of host-mediated antitumor activity in mice by B-glucan obtained from Grifola frondosa (Maitake)." (*Chemical and Pharmaceutical Bulletin* 35:262-270).

Blackburn, George L., and Wang, Katherine A. 2007. "Dietary fat reduction and breast cancer outcome: results from the Women's Intervention Nutrition Study (WINS)." (*Am J Clin Nutr*; 86(suppl):878S– 81S).

Boothby, Lisa, A., Doering, Paul L., and Kipersztok, Simon 2004. "Bioidentical hormone therapy: a review." (*Menopause: The Journal of The North American Menopause Society* Vol. 11, No. 3, pp. 356-367).

Bosetti, C., Spertini, L., Parpinel, M., Gnagnarella, P., Lagiou, P., Negri, E., Franceschi, S., Montell, M., Peterson, J., Dwyer, J., Giacosa, A., and La Vecchia, C. 2005. "Flavonoids and breast cancer risk in Italy." (*Cancer Epidemiol Biomarkers Prev.* Apr;14(4):805-8. Review).

Caygill, C.P., Charlett, A., Hill, M.J. 1996. "Fat, fish, fish oil and cancer." (*Br J Cancer.* Jul;74(1):159-64).

Choi J.A., et al. 2001. "Induction of cell cycle arrest and apoptosis in human breast cancer cells by quercitin." (*International Journal of Oncology.* 19(4): 837-44, Oct.).

Elena, P., Moiseeva, Gabriela M., Almeida, George D., Jones, D., and Manson, Margaret M. 2007. "Extended treatment with physiologic concentrations of dietary phytochemicals results in altered gene expression, reduced growth, and apoptosis of cancer cells." (*Mol Cancer Ther* 2007;6(11):3071–9).

Fink, B. N., Steck, S.E., Wolff, M.S., Britton, J.A., Kabat, G.C., Schroeder, J.C., Teitelbaum, S.L., Neugut, A.I., and Gammon, M.D. 2007. "Dietary flavonoid intake and breast cancer risk among women on Long Island." (*Am J Epidemiol.* 2007, Mar 1; 165(5):514-23).

Fink, B.N., Steck, S.E., Wolff, M.S., Britton, J.A., Kabat, G.C., Gaudet, M.M., Abrahamson, P.E., Bell, P., Schroeder, J.C., Teitelbaum, S.L., Neugut, A.I., Gammon, M.D. 2007. "Dietary Flavonoid Intake and Breast Cancer Survival among Women on Long Island." (*Cancer Epidemiol Biomarkers Prev.* Nov; 16 (11):2285-92).

Fleischauer, A.T., and Arab, L. 2001. ""Garlic and cancer: a critical review of the epidemiologic literature." (*J. Nutrition* 131: 1032S-1040S).

Grzanna, R., et al. 2004. "Ginger extract inhibits beta-amyloid peptide-induced cytokine and chemokine expression in cultured THP-1 monocytes." (*Journal of Alternative & Complementary Medicine.* 10(6): 1009-13, Dec.).

Guha, N., et al. 2009. "Soy isoflavones and risk of cancer recurrence in a cohort of breast cancer survivors: the Life after Cancer Epidemiology study." (*Breast Cancer Res Treat* 118: 395-405).

Ikekawa, T., Uehara, N., Y., Maeda, Y., M., Nakanishi, M., Fukuoka, F. 1969. "Twenty years of Studies on Antitumor Activities of Mushrooms." (*Cancer Research* 29, 734-735).

John, Esther, M., Schwartz, Gary G., Dreon, Darlene M., and Koo, Jocelyn 1999. "Vitamin D and Breast Cancer Risk: The NHANES I Epidemiologic Follow-up Study, 1971–1975 to 1992." (*Cancer Epidemiology, Biomarkers & Prevention* Vol. 8, 399–406, May).

Kuo, Y.C., Lin, C. Y., Tsai, W. J. and Wu, C. L., Chen, C. F., & Shiao, M. S. 1994. "Growth inhibitors against tumor cells in *Cordyceps sinensis* other than cordycepin and polysaccharides." (*Cancer-Investigation.* 12(6): 611-5).

Kuriki, Kiyonori; Hirose, Kaoru; Wakai, Kenjo; Matsuo, Keitaro; Ito, Hidemi; Suzuki, Takeshi; Hiraki, Akio; Saito, Toshiko; Iwata, Hiroji; Tatematsu, Masae, and Kazuo Tajima, Kazuo. 2007. "Breast cancer risk and erythrocyte compositions of n-3 highly unsaturated fatty acids in Japanese." (*Int. J. Cancer:* 121, 377–385).

Kushi, Lawrence; Byers, Tim; Doyle, Colleen; Bandera, Elisa V., McCullough, Marji; Gansler, Ted; Andrews, Kimberly S., Thun, Michael J., and The American Cancer Society, 2006; Nutrition and Physical Activity Guidelines Advisory Committee. 2006. "American Cancer Society Guidelines on Nutrition and Physical Activity for Cancer Prevention: Reducing the Risk of Cancer With Healthy Food Choices and Physical Activity." (*CA Cancer J Clin*; 56;254-281).

Limer, Jane L., and Speirs, Valerie 2004. "Review: Phyto-estrogens and breast cancer chemoprevention." *Breast Cancer Res* 2004, 6:119-127).

Low Dog, T., Riley, D., and Carter, T. 2001. "Traditional and Alternative Therapies for Breast Cancer." (*Alternative Therapies in Health & Medicine*, May/Jun, Vol. 7, Issue 3, p36.).

Maizes, Victoria 2005. "Reducing the Risk of Breast Cancer: Nutritional Strategies." (*EXPLORE*, March, Vol. 1, No. 2).

Messina, M.J. 1999. "Legumes and Soybeans: overview of their nutritional profiles and health effects." (*American Journal of Clinical Nutrition*; 70(suppl):439S-50S).

Michael, J., Wargovich, Cynthia; Woods, Destiny, M., Hollis, and Mary E. Zander 2001. "Herbals, Cancer Prevention and Health." (*J. Nutr.* 131: 3034S–3036S.

Milner, J.A. 2001. "A historical perspective on garlic and cancer." (*J. Nutrition* 131: 1027S-1031S).

Milner, J.A. 2001. "Mechanisms by which garlic and allyl sulfur compounds suppress carcinogen bioactivation. Garlic and carcinogenesis." (*Adv. Exp. Med. Biol* 492: 69-81).

Mizuno, T, H. Saito, T., Nishitoba, & Kawagishi, H. 1995. "Antitumor active substances from mushrooms." (*Food Reviews International* 111: 23-61. Marcel Dekker, New York).

Nanba, H., 1995. "Activity of Maitake D-Fraction to Inhibit Carcinogenesis and Metastasis." (*Annals of the New York Academy of Sciences*, vol. 768: 243-245).

NCI Fact Sheet: "Red Wine and Cancer Prevention": *http://www.cancer. gov/cancertopics/factsheet/red-wine-and-cancer-prevention*

NCI Fact Sheet: "Tea and Cancer Prevention": *http://www.cancer.gov/ cancertopics/factsheet/tea-and-cancer-prevention*

Peterson, J., Lagiou, P., Samoli, E., Lagiou, A., Katsouyanni, K., La Vecchia, C., Dwyer, J. and Trichopoulos, D. (2003). "Flavonoid intake and breast cancer risk: a case-control study in Greece." (*Br J Cancer.* Oct 6; 89(7):1255-9).

Qin, Li-Qiang, et al. 2006. "Soyfood Intake in the Prevention of Breast Cancer Risk in Women: A Meta-analysis of Observational Epidemiological Studies." (*J Nutr Sci Vitaminol,* 52, 428-436).

Questions and Answers about Beta Carotene Chemoprevention Trials. 1997. National Cancer Institute Fact Sheet.

Qinghui, Meng; Itzhak, D., Goldberg, Eliot M., Rosen and Saijun, Fan. 2000. "Inhibitory effects of Indole-3-carbinol on invasion and migration in human breast cancer cells." (*Breast Cancer Research and Treatment* 63: 147–152).

Rietveld, A., Wiseman, S. 2003. "Antioxidant Effects of Tea: Evidence from Human Clinical Trials." (*J. Nutr.* 133: 3285S-3292S).

Sengupta, A., Ghosh, S., Bhattacharjee, S. 2004. "Allium Vegetables in Cancer Prevention: An Overview." (*Asian Pacific J Cancer Prev*, 5, 237-245).

Shannon, Jackilen; King, Irena B., Moshofsky, Rachel; Lampe, Johanna W., Gao, Dao Li; Ray, Roberta M., and Thomas, David B. "Erythrocyte fatty acids and breast cancer risk: a case-control study in Shanghai, China." (*American Journal of Clinical Nutrition*, Vol. 85, No. 4, 1090-1097, April 2007).

Shannon, J., King, I.B., Moshofsky, R., Lampe, J.W., Li, Gao D., Ray, R.M., Thomas, D.B. 2007. "Erythrocyte fatty acids and breast cancer risk: a case-control study in Shanghai, China." (*Am J Clin Nutr.* 2007 Apr; 85(4):1090-7).

Singletary, K., MacDonald, C., Wallig, M. 1996. "Inhibition by rosemary and carnosol of 7,12-dimethylbenz[a]anthracene (DMBA)-induced rat mammary tumorigenesis and in vivo DMBA-DNA adduct formation." (*Cancer Lett.* Jun 24;104(1):43-8).

Somasundaram, S., et al., 2002. "Dietary Curcumin Inhibits Chemotherapy-induced Apoptosis in Models of Human Breast Cancer." (*Cancer Research* 62, 3868–3875, July 1).

Tapiero, H., Nguyen Ba, G., Couvreur, P., Tew, K.D. 2002. "Polyunsaturated fatty acids (PUFA) and eicosanoids in human health and pathologies." (*Biomed Pharmacother* 56, 215–222).

Verma, S. P., Salamone, E., and Goldin, B. 1997. "Curcumin and Genistein, Plant Natural Products Show Synergistic Inhibitory Effects on the Growth of Human Breast Cancer MCF-7 Cells Induced by Estrogenic Pesticides." (*Biochemical and Biophysical Research Communications* 233, 692–696).

World Cancer Research Fund / American Institute for Cancer Research. 2007. "Food, Nutrition, Physical Activity, and the Prevention of Cancer: a Global Perspective." (Washington DC: AICR).

World Cancer Research Fund / American Institute for Cancer Research. 2009. "Policy and Action for Cancer Prevention. Food, Nutrition, and Physical Activity: a Global Perspective." (Washington DC: AICR).

Zhou, Jin-Rong; Li, Linglin, and Pan, Weijun 2007. "Dietary soy and tea combinations for prevention of breast and prostate cancers by targeting metabolic syndrome elements in mice." (*Am J Clin Nutr*; 86(suppl): 882S–8S).

Index

Acknowledgments

A little over 10 years ago, my wife Gail challenged my assumption that everything I needed to know about health was contained in the biomedical model. Her prodding started my thinking outside that little box and ignited the whole process that resulted in this book. I would not be the same doctor, writer, teacher, or person today were it not for her insatiable appetite for growth and change. She has all of my love and gratitude.

The faculty, staff, and fellows of the Arizona Center for Integrative Medicine have been a constant source of encouragement to me and have challenged me to expand the scope of my medical practice, teaching and writing. They have all been my teachers. Of the many, I must mention a few faculty members who especially embodied for me the new way of seeing health and medicine which now defines my practice and teaching: Howard Silverman, Victoria Maizes, Randy Horwitz, Tieraona Low Dog, and Andrew Weil.

A special word of thanks to my mentor and teacher, Dr. Andrew Weil. His encyclopedic grasp of the role of foods in disease prevention continues to inspire me, as does his ongoing mission to change the face of the healthcare system by bringing Integrative Medicine into the mainstream of medical education.

It's one thing to write a manuscript and quite another to publish a book. It could not have happened without the guidance and support of my editors Danielle Wong Moores and John Maling, my book shepherd Judith Briles, book design and cover art from Nick Zelinger, and internet marketing guidance from Rana Burr.

And finally, when I stop long enough to sit quietly and reflect, I know that all of my inspiration and energy is a gift from my Creator, through whatever human hands it may pass. In the words which J.S. Bach chose to sign his musical masterpieces: "Soli Deo Gloria."

Robert Pendergrast, MD, MPH
Fall, 2010

About the Author

Robert Pendergrast, M.D. is a graduate of Furman University, the Medical College of Georgia and the John Hopkins University School of Hygiene and Public Health. He is a Fellow of the American Academy of Pediatrics, certified by the American Society of Clinical Hypnosis and a graduate of the Fellowship at the Center for Integrative Medicine at the University of Arizona. Dr. Pendergrast has taught medical students and residents in Pediatrics for over 20 years. In 2004, he was voted Educator of the Year by students at the Medical Center of Georgia and continues his passion as an educator on the faculty there.

He is a sought after speaker at medical education meetings for professionals. With his wife Gail, he does workshops for the public, providing empowerment for individuals to take charge of their own health. Additionally, he has a consulting private practice for all ages where he combines his love of nutritional medicine, clinical hypnotherapy and herbal medicine.

Dr. Pendergrast can be reached for consultations and speaking engagements through his website:

www.Holistic-Medicine-MD.com

Order Form

To order additional copies of this book via U.S. Mail, please remove or copy this page and return the completed form to:

Penstokes Press • P.O. Box 7798 • North Augusta, SC 29861
803-426-1421 • fax 803-426-1423

Send to (please print):

_____
Name

_____
Address

_____
City

_____
State   Zip   Country

_____
Email

Breast Cancer: Reduce Your Risk with Foods You Love – Per copy: $24.00

U.S. Postage & Handling – Per copy: $5.00

Book Subtotal _____
        $24.00 each (U.S.) includes $5/copy shipping and handling

Total enclosed with order: _____

Please pay by check or money order, payable to Penstokes Press.

Credit Card Method of Payment:

___Check   ___Cash   ___Credit Card (Visa, MC, Discover) # of copies: _____

Credit Card number _____   Exp Date: _____

CVV # (3 digits on back): _____

Shipping Address: _____

City, State, Zip: _____

Phone: _____   E-mail: _____

Street address #, Zip Code of billing address of card (if different):

_____

Order Form

To order additional copies of this book via U.S. Mail, please remove or copy this page and return the completed form to:

Penstokes Press • P.O. Box 7798 • North Augusta, SC 29861
803-426-1421 • fax 803-426-1423

Send to (please print):

_____
Name

_____
Address

_____
City

_____
State   Zip   Country

_____
Email

Breast Cancer: Reduce Your Risk with Foods You Love – Per copy: $24.00

U.S. Postage & Handling – Per copy: $5.00

Book Subtotal _____
       $24.00 each (U.S.) includes $5/copy shipping and handling

Total enclosed with order: _____

Please pay by check or money order, payable to Penstokes Press.

Credit Card Method of Payment:

___Check   ___Cash   ___Credit Card (Visa, MC, Discover) # of copies: ____

Credit Card number _____   Exp Date: _____

CVV # (3 digits on back): _____

Shipping Address: _____

City, State, Zip: _____

Phone: _____   E-mail: _____

Street address #, Zip Code of billing address of card (if different):

_____

www.PenstokesPress.com